Praise for *The Inflammation Spectrum*

"Will Cole is one of the most curious and compassionate health practitioners we have worked with at Goop. In *The Inflammation Spectrum*, he shares his helpful, simple-to-follow toolbox, along with his compelling and empowering perspective on reclaiming and optimizing your health."

—GWYNETH PALTROW, founder of Goop and
New York Times–bestselling author of *The Clean Plate*

"Dr. Cole has done a terrific job highlighting the role of inflammation as a pivotal player in a broad swath of our most pervasive and tenacious health issues. Focusing on chronic inflammation and the lifestyle modifications that can facilitate its resolution is fundamental for regaining and preserving health, and these goals are wonderfully achieved in *The Inflammation Spectrum*."

—DAVID PERLMUTTER, MD, FACN, *New York Times*–
bestselling author of *Grain Brain* and *Brain Maker*

"*The Inflammation Spectrum* is the book we have all been needing. Just as he did with *Ketotarian*, Dr. Will Cole wows us again by shedding new light on inflammation with a fresh solution. With this book, you'll not only learn how inflammation impacts your health, you'll also discover the specific foods your body loves and hates, to start healing your health problems—no guessing needed."

—ALEJANDRO JUNGER, MD, *New York Times*–
bestselling author of *Clean Gut* and *Clean Eats*

"*The Inflammation Spectrum* is for anyone who is fed up with fad diets. My colleague Dr. Will Cole has used his years of functional medicine experience to brilliantly lay out a plan that anyone can use to feel and look their best. Achieve food freedom by finally discovering which foods are truly optimal for your body and how that can manifest into sustainable, lifelong wellness."

—MARK HYMAN, MD, director, Cleveland Clinic Center for
Functional Medicine, and *New York Times*–bestselling author of *Food*

"Inflammation is such a hot topic in the wellness world, and *The Inflammation Spectrum* finally provides us with the answers to all of our questions. Dr. Will Cole explains how inflammation exists on a continuum and shows you how to discover where you are on that spectrum. If you've ever been confused about your health, this is the book to read to start making positive changes naturally, through delicious food medicines."

—JOSH AXE, DNM, DC, CNS, bestselling author of
Keto Diet and *Eat Dirt*

"Dr. Will Cole is a go-to expert on all things functional medicine for my clients' health problems. *The Inflammation Spectrum* makes it easy to find which foods work best for your body. He takes it one step further by giving you the tools to apply that knowledge to your life in a very practical way through finding out which foods your body loves. This is grace-based eating at its best."

—KELLY LEVEQUE, celebrity nutritionist and author of *Body Love*

"Inflammation is the root of all evil when it comes to health. It's a serious problem that many of us are living with and we don't even know it! With Dr. Will Cole's *The Inflammation Spectrum*, there's finally a program and a protocol to put us on a path to fight inflammation and achieve optimal health and happiness."

—JASON WACHOB, founder and co-CEO, MindBodyGreen, and
author of *Wellth*

"If you could summarize what is at the root cause of all diseases of civilization, it would come down to inflammation, hands down. In *The Inflammation Spectrum*, Dr. Will Cole offers up his invaluable clinical wisdom on how to nourish yourself to keep the fires of inflammation at bay. This book will help you put out the fire that's keeping you fat and sick with a whole food–based ketogenic diet that's tailor-made for you."

—JIMMY MOORE, bestselling author of *Keto Clarity* and co-author
of *The Complete Guide to Fasting*

"Healers like Will Cole are the great promise—and future—of preventative medicine. In his practice, Dr. Cole offers highly individuated and intuitive care that puts you on a wellness spectrum—with the goal of keeping you on the vital end. In today's high-stress world, where autoimmune disease runs rampant among women, he brings a much-needed focus to stopping chronic illness before it takes hold."

—ELISE LOEHNEN, chief content officer, Goop

"Finally! *All* the smart questions you *want* your health practitioner to ask! My esteemed colleague Dr. Will Cole gets it right with *The Inflammation Spectrum*. As a gut-health expert, I know the root of most chronic inflammation is in the gut, and how individualized, tailored prescriptions for health through diet, recipes, and meal plans can change lives. Dr. Cole's book features functional medicine–based quizzes that can help everyone be a sleuth to discover their unique inflammation and health profile."

—VINCENT PEDRE, MD, bestselling author of *Happy Gut*

"In *The Inflammation Spectrum*, Dr. Will Cole eloquently explains the root cause of health problems and offers a fun, innovative plan to begin lowering inflammation and reclaiming optimal wellness."

—TERRY WAHLS, MD, IFMCP, author of *The Wahls Protocol*

"Once again my friend Dr. Will Cole has created a means of education around a topic that is so controllable but often neglected.... As a chef devoted to changing the world through food, I am excited for you to enjoy the epic education that is found within the following pages."

—DAN CHURCHILL, author of *DudeFood*

"In *The Inflammation Spectrum*, my friend Dr. Will Cole brings love and grace back to wellness. Doing away with dieting dogma, Will teaches us how to find out which foods make us feel our very best."

—KELLY RUTHERFORD, actress

"Dr. Will Cole does an amazing job of showing us how inflammation plays a vital role in shaping our health. He brilliantly explains the roots of chronic health problems and provides hope and innovative, practical ways to overcome inflammation and come out on the other side with restored health for a thriving life."

—DHRU PUROHIT, host of *The Broken Brain*

THE
INFLAMMATION
SPECTRUM

THE
INFLAMMATION
SPECTRUM

Find Your Food Triggers
and Reset Your System

DR. WILL COLE

with Eve Adamson

Avery
an imprint of Penguin Random House
New York

AVERY

an imprint of Penguin Random House LLC

penguinrandomhouse.com

First trade paperback edition 2022

Most Avery books are available at special quantity discounts for bulk purchase for sales promotions, premiums, fund-raising, and educational needs. Special books or book excerpts also can be created to fit specific needs. For details, write SpecialMarkets@penguinrandomhouse.com.

Illustrations by Michael Weaver

The Library of Congress has catalogued the hardcover edition as follows:

Names: Cole, Will (Functional medicine expert). | Adamson, Eve, author.
Title: The inflammation spectrum : find your food triggers and reset your system / Will Cole, Eve Adamson.
Description: New York : Avery, 2019. | Includes bibliographical references and index.
Identifiers: LCCN 2019015847 | ISBN 9780735220089 (hardback) | ISBN 9780735220096 (ebook)
Subjects: LCSH: Inflammation—Popular works. | Inflammation—Diet therapy—Popular works. | Inflammation—Diet therapy—Recipes. | BISAC: HEALTH & FITNESS / Diets. | MEDICAL / Diet Therapy.
Classification: LCC RB131.C652 2019 | DDC 616/.0473—dc23
LC record available at https://lccn.loc.gov/2019015847

ISBN (paperback) 9780735220102
ISBN (ebook) 9780735220096

Printed in the United States of America
4th Printing

Book design by Lorie Pagnozzi

To Amber, Solomon, and Shiloh:
When I look at you, I see the heart of God—
boundless love, grace, and acceptance.
May these qualities permeate the pages of this book.

CONTENTS

Introduction   1

CHAPTER ONE
ANTICIP8: How Bio-Individuality Determines
What Your Body Loves and Hates   13

CHAPTER TWO
INVESTIG8: Discover Your Personalized
Inflammation Profile   32

CHAPTER THREE
INCORPOR8: Your Track and Your Toolbox   56

CHAPTER FOUR
INITI8: Transitioning into the Elimination Phase   83

CHAPTER FIVE
ELIMIN8 OR CORE4: Cool Inflammation
and Heal   106

CHAPTER SIX
DEDIC8: Your Anti-Inflammatory Cookbook   192

CHAPTER SEVEN
REINTEGR8: Testing Your Old Favorites   256

CHAPTER EIGHT
CRE8: How to Design Your New, Personalized
Food and Life Plan   282

Acknowledgments   293
Notes   295
Index   307

THE
INFLAMMATION
SPECTRUM

INTRODUCTION

Your body is alive because of brilliant biochemistry. As a vast sixty thousand miles of blood vessels run through you, your body is producing 25 million new cells each and every second. There are more intricate connections in your brain than there are stars in the galaxy. In fact, the trillions of diverse cells in your body were actually formed from the same carbon, nitrogen, and oxygen in the stars that shone brightly billions of years ago. In other words, you are literally made of stardust. While these trillions of cells all have their own unique purpose, they also have one thing in common: They exist so that you may thrive. This is how intricately and profoundly special you are. For eons, throughout time and human existence, no one—not one person—has ever had your unique confluence of genes, biochemistry, and beauty, until you.

For each of us, every food we eat instructs our biochemistry. Every meal, every bite of food we take, constantly and dynamically influences how we feel. But because no one else is you, there are no hard-and-fast rules that will reveal one universal list of good and bad foods. The foods that work well for someone else may not be right for you and your unique biochemistry. This book is just for you. It is your personal guide to finding out which foods *your body* loves, hates, and needs to feel great.

As a functional medicine practitioner, I specialize in helping people learn the language of their bodies so they can discover exactly what they are doing (or not doing) during the course of each

> **What foods cause inflammation for you? What foods are nutritious and beneficial for you?**

day that may be helping or hurting their unique biochemistry. I have helped thousands of patients lose weight and regain vitality by teaching them how to tap into their own deep internal wisdom. What foods cause inflammation for you? What foods are nutritious and beneficial for you? Your body knows. Your diet should be exclusive to you, but how do you know the right foods for you? How do you learn to hear what your body is telling you so that you can nourish it and flourish?

THE AGE OF INFLAMMATION

Discovering your unique diet is important for optimizing health, but there is an even more important reason to intervene into the dietary and lifestyle habits that don't serve you. There is a storm brewing. Clouds are gathering on the horizon and they're coming our way. It is the storm of inflammation. The signs are already upon us. A shocking 60 percent of American adults have a chronic disease, and 40 percent have two or more chronic diseases.[1] Today someone will have a heart attack every 40 seconds,[2] cancer is the second leading cause of death worldwide,[3] 50 million Americans have an autoimmune disease,[4] and almost half the population of the United States has either prediabetes or diabetes.[5]

Brain health problems are also on the rise. Around 20 percent of adults have a diagnosable mental disorder.[6] Depression is now the leading cause of disability around the world. Around 1 in 5 American children ages three to seventeen (about 15 million kids) have a diagnosable mental, emotional, or behavioral disorder. Serious depression is worsening, especially among teens, with the suicide rate among teen girls reaching a forty-year high.[7] Anxiety impacts more than 40 million Americans, and Alzheimer's disease is the sixth leading cause of death in the United States. Since 1979, deaths due to brain disease have increased by 66 percent in men and a whopping 92 percent in women.[8] One in 59 children are now on the autism spectrum.[9]

Why is this happening? There is one underlying commonality between all these different health problems—one link that binds these atrocities. Every single one of these health problems is inflammatory in nature. Sadly, this is the age of inflammation.

What is the top, and oftentimes the only, option given by mainstream medicine for these chronic inflammatory health problems? Pharmaceutical drugs. A staggering 81 percent of us take at least one medication a day. But are all these pharmaceutical "fixes" actually helping?

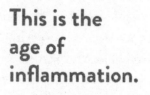

This is the age of inflammation.

We spend more money than any other country on health care,[10] yet our life expectancy is shorter, obesity is more widespread, and the rate of maternal and infant death is higher than in any other industrialized nation in the world. Prescription drugs, in fact, are now said to kill more people than heroin and cocaine combined.[11] Certainly some people are alive because of medications, and modern medicine has brought us amazing advancements in emergency care. But who can look at these statistics and conclude that the mainstream approach to chronic health problems is effective or sustainable?

But why do we have to choose between modern medicine and getting healthy? There is a time and place for lifesaving conventional medicine. For every health decision we make, I believe we should ask, "What is the most effective option for me that causes the fewest side effects?" For some, medications fit this criterion, but for many others, they do not. Medications are not the most effective option for many people with many different kinds of health problems, even though drugs are often the only option conventional medicine has to offer. And most modern pharmaceutical medications have a long list of potential side effects (you've seen those drug commercials). How can we even call this modern system *health care*? There is very little *health* or *care* in mainstream medicine today. "Disease management" or "sick care" would be more descriptive.

Patients come to see me or consult with me online from all over the world for many reasons, but one of the most common is that conventional medicine has not provided solutions or relief for their chronic health issues. These health problems can vary widely, but what I see most often are cases of digestive distress, autoimmune conditions, hormone imbalances, persistent anxiety or depression, weight loss resistance, and unrelenting fatigue. My patients have a desire to address the cause of an issue rather than just masking it with pharmaceuticals that often have side effects just as bad or worse than the symptoms they are supposed to relieve.

When patients come to see me, I talk and listen to them extensively. I give them several questionnaires (which I've adapted for this book) to really investigate where their symptoms are rooted and where they are most vulnerable to inflammation. Then, unlike conventional doctors, who are taught to follow a model of matching symptoms to a diagnosis and a corresponding medication, I work with my patients to discover the underlying facets of their chronic health issues. I'm not just interested in "How do we stop the symptoms?" I am also interested in "How do we find and fix the root cause of the symptoms so they resolve on their own?" To me, this is a more sensible and direct approach, because who ultimately has health problems due to a pharmaceutical deficiency?

This is an important, even critical, difference between the way I practice functional medicine (more about that shortly) and the way conventionally trained doctors practice. You've probably heard the quote from Hippocrates: "Let food be thy medicine and medicine thy food." How far have we strayed when the father of modern medicine's words are considered radical and threatening to mainstream medicine? In conventional medicine, food is an afterthought, if it is thought of at all.

But food should not be an afterthought. Food is powerful medicine. The problem is, you aren't likely to get much information about this kind of "prescription" from your conventionally trained doctor. Today in U.S. medical schools, students on average receive only about nineteen hours of nutrition education over their four years of school,[12] and only 29 percent of U.S. medical schools even offer med students the recommended twenty-five hours of nutrition education.[13] A study in the *International Journal of Adolescent Medicine and Health* assessed the basic nutrition and health knowledge of medical school graduates entering a pediatric residency program and found that they were able to correctly answer an average of just 52 percent of the eighteen questions. In short, most doctors would fail a basic nutrition exam because they simply don't have the necessary training in this field.[14]

It's ironic that nutrition is such a low priority for mainstream medicine, since a startling 80 percent of the most common chronic diseases (heart disease, cancer, autoimmunity, diabetes) are almost always preventable and reversible with lifestyle choices.[15] If almost all of the chronic health problems we face as a world today are preventable, reversible, improvable, manageable, or overcome-able naturally, why would we settle for anything less? Just because something is common doesn't mean it's normal. Chronic inflammatory health problems and a growing prescription list are certainly ubiquitous, but they are definitely *not* normal.

FUNCTIONAL MEDICINE: THE FUTURE OF CARING HEALTH

Functional medicine is an emerging mode of health care that differs from conventional medicine. Functional medicine practitioners consider food and lifestyle medicine to be primary modes of health restoration, rather than prioritizing pharmaceutical intervention as the first (and sometimes only) option for managing chronic disease. Because of this, those of us experienced in this method of health care have extensive training in the potent effects of both food and lifestyle. We don't have a problem with medication when it is needed, but the focus is on the bigger picture of a patient's life because we know that what you eat and how you live directly influence your health and wellness. Since conventional doctors don't typically have the training to guide people in lifestyle changes, people who depend on their doctors for help (especially those whose symptoms don't fit the standard model) are often left with nothing but unresolved health issues and a growing list of prescription medicines and their side effects. Functional medicine offers another way, one in which food leads the charge.

One of the most powerful methods I teach to my patients about how to begin taking control of their health and getting to the root of their problems is how to use their meals as medicine. We start there, almost always, because every bite of food you eat is either feeding health or fighting it. Every meal is an opportunity to nourish wellness or erode it—to move you further along the spectrum toward increased inflammation, or in the direction of calming inflammation and improving your symptoms and overall health. There is no neutral food, no Switzerland meal.

There is no neutral food.

But here's the tricky part: The foods

that move *you* closer to or further away from health may be completely different from the foods that do that for anyone else. We're all somewhere on a spectrum based on the degree of inflammation we have in our systems—but what moves us in one direction or the other is anything but one-size-fits-all. The reason I practice functional medicine is that it puts individuality first and foremost. Functional medicine practitioners understand that no diet or prescription will work for everyone—even those with the same symptoms—because too many other factors influence the way symptoms present themselves, and any given symptom could have many different possible causes.

But how do you know what foods to choose? How do you know what foods and lifestyle habits are boosting your health and which might be worsening your symptoms, contributing to your weight loss resistance, draining your energy, or causing you pain? The truth is that there is only one best and proven way to do this, without question and without competition: by doing an elimination diet.

THE POWER AND PURPOSE OF AN ELIMINATION DIET

To date, no lab tests can reliably and consistently detect your food intolerances and sensitivities. No lab test can tell you definitively that this or that food will cause symptoms for you in any manner close to the proven results you can get from doing a carefully planned and executed elimination diet. An elimination diet can precisely pinpoint the exact foods that are inflammatory for any individual. The problem with most elimination diets, however—the ones doctors and dietitians have used for decades—is that they are boring, generic, and unsustainable, even over the temporary time for which they are prescribed. And an accurate elimination diet must be longer than a week. You could end up feeling like you are in food prison!

But it doesn't have to be like that.

The elimination diet I give to my patients is different. I know from years of experience that not everybody is likely to be sensitive or reactive to everything, and in fact people with certain symptoms are *more likely* to be intolerant of certain types of foods, as well as to benefit from certain types of food medicine. Knowing and acting on this truth can make the practice of an elimination diet more personalized, sustainable, and interesting.

The fresh elimination diet plan you'll find in this book is designed to be personalized, rather than based on some generic idea of an unhealthy person. It takes into consideration the most bothersome symptoms and the greatest concerns and adds customized recommendations based on your unique symptom profile. It also goes one step further, including not just foods but lifestyle habits to add and to eliminate, in order to improve health from all corners, even beyond food. My elimination diet is targeted specifically to *you*—no matter who you are, where you live, or what you like to eat and do. It is more fun and interesting and more likely to keep you engaged in the process, because the truth is, an elimination diet won't tell you much if you don't finish it.

The questionnaires and quizzes I have designed for you in this book will help you define your areas of concern, and the tools, tips, and specialty information allow you to DIY your way back to health. You'll find:

■ Valuable information about where you fall on the inflammation spectrum, which will determine which of the two elimination tracks you should follow.

■ Customized medicinal foods and therapies to address your symptoms at their source, neatly organized in your personalized toolbox.

- Step-by-step guidance through the process so you are never unsure about what to do.

- Instructions for creating a personalized life list of foods that are most nourishing and healing for you.

- Best of all, a new level of body wisdom and perspective on how to live well going forward, all fully customized according to your needs, goals, desires, and dreams.

You have never experienced anything like this in a book before.

While I do believe there are some foods that aren't good for anyone (I wouldn't recommend junk foods with additives like high-fructose corn syrup or trans-fat-containing foods to anyone, for example), within the world of whole, real foods, the ultimate diet for you really is a matter of your unique biochemistry, genetics, personal preferences, and gut microbiome balance. I have seen the "healthiest" real food work wonderfully well for one person and trigger inflammation in the next, and the plan in this book is your key to finding your personal food prescription.

That means you can finally end your frustrating search for the "perfect diet." I'm never going to tell you that everyone should go vegan or keto to be healthy. I'm never going to make broad, sweeping statements declaring that everyone should eat only plants every day or assume that everyone should be a carnivore. Even though my first book, *Ketotarian*, is a plant-based ketogenic food guide, we are all ultimately different, which is why I made *Ketotarian* with different vegan, vegetarian, and pescatarian keto options. Even within the paradigm of plant-based, keto, or any other way of eating, the optimal food choices within those diets vary from person to person. If you like to eat a certain way, that's fine! But the actual foods you choose require a little bit of self-knowledge, and this book will help you get that knowledge and act on it.

This is the beauty of *The Inflammation Spectrum*. I will help you to discover the one way of eating that is right for *you*. Whether you prefer to eat plant-based, ketogenic, paleo, or Mediterranean, or you eat whatever the heck you want, you can achieve better health and slide back down the inflammation spectrum to a place of radiant wellness by finding out which foods work for you and which foods do not in a way that is pleasurable, nutritious, delicious, and most of all, doable. I believe food and wellness should be fun and magical and I try to convey that to my patients and in my writings: *Ketotarian* was the alchemy between plant-based and keto diets. *The Inflammation Spectrum* is the transmutation of food confusion into food freedom.

We in functional medicine know that health is a complex and dynamic force. Someone who appears to eat a junky diet may have glowing health because of the positive influences of a low-stress lifestyle, a supportive social group, and lots of exercise. Someone else may eat like a health rock star, throwing back kombucha and kale salads on a daily basis, but may be withering from loneliness or the crushing stress that can trigger serious health issues. Even if we limit our focus to food alone, one person's health food may be inflammatory for another person—that kale you eat may give someone else digestive issues, and the dark chocolate your friend seems to enjoy without consequence may give you a migraine. This is why dieting dogma is antiquated and has no place here.

Instead, those of us in the functional medicine community look at people within the context of their environments, to see how well they are functioning and to assess the big picture: what they eat, how they live, and how every aspect of their existence may impact them physically, emotionally, and spiritually. My goal is to get you actively moving toward health by helping you discover the foods, lifestyle habits, and other therapies that best nourish and meet your individual needs in the context of *your* life. This is your big picture approach, and it begins with taking a good close look at how you live.

With its personalized profiling, customized elimination process, and clear, organized reintegration of foods, the *Inflammation Spectrum* program can help anyone discover what may be best and worst for them to eat, take, try, and do. It resolves the internal battle between lifestyle choices and health needs by answering that ultimate question: "What do *I* need?" Let's illuminate your personal path to health.

1

ANTICIP8: HOW BIO-INDIVIDUALITY DETERMINES WHAT YOUR BODY LOVES AND HATES

We all have the same rough outlines, the same external appendages and internal organs, the same basic processes happening within. Our hearts beat. Our blood travels throughout our veins and arteries. Our muscles flex and extend. Our bones hold us up. Yet the subtle fluctuations in each body's biochemistry are unique to the individual.

Some of this variability has to do with genetics (the unique set of variations in your DNA) and epigenetics (how your lifestyle and environment influence the expression of your genes). Some of it has to do with the balance and diversity of your gut bacteria, the regulation of your immune system, the fluctuations in your hormones, and your level of inflammation at any given moment. In fact, what causes inflammation in you may be completely different from what causes inflammation in someone else, and how inflammation affects your health and functioning is also unique.

All these things and more are interconnected and mutually influential, creating the complex and ever-changing miracle that is distinctively you. You are different from anyone else, in a trillion tiny ways. You have your unique strengths and challenges. There are everyday factors (foods, activities, and thoughts) that make you feel great and others that make you feel lousy. You also likely have your own symptom set—maybe you are prone to migraines, fatigue, joint pain, rashes, or anxiety. Maybe you tend to have digestive problems, your hormones are imbalanced, or you have trouble losing weight. Each one of these issues is related to your health and is likely influenced in many ways, not just by your genetics and microbiome but by what you eat, how you move, how you live your life—even how you think.

Everything you do either increases your health or decreases your health—and in many cases, that means *everything* you do either increases inflammation or decreases it. But *what exactly* does what for you is unique to you. What makes you healthier or less healthy is not necessarily the same as what makes someone else healthier or less healthy. What a beautiful puzzle you are!

This puzzle, with its uniquely shaped pieces, is called bio-individuality. Recognizing bio-individuality is one of the foundational aspects of functional medicine, and as a functional medicine practitioner, I know that bio-individuality is the single most powerful source of information about you and your health. I see bio-individuality playing out in my patients every day. By the time they find their way to me, most of my patients are already eating dramatically better than the standard Western diet. They are already well-read in wellness and have been on their health journey for a while when they discover functional medicine. No matter what diet they might be on, they mostly eat real whole food. Yet despite their healthy intentions, they all come to me with some level of health dysfunction. Part of the reason is that the diet they are eating is not working optimally *for them*.

The diet industry relies on the notion that some diets will work very well for some people. This is why you see so many books, articles, and blog posts about the next "miracle diet," *the one thing that finally helped*. But that "one thing" someone found only worked because it just happened to be right for that person—it happened to be bio-individually appropriate *for them*. Have you noticed the fine print in those television ads that reads, "Results not typical"? If others try to replicate those results, they will likely be unsuccessful because their *one thing* is probably something different—maybe dramatically different. Maybe the exact opposite of whatever is being advertised. Their puzzle has completely different pieces.

One person's food medicine is another person's food problem. Bio-individuality is the reason. If you are not aware of your intolerances or sensitivities, you may unknowingly be eating a food, maybe even daily, that is aggravating your symptoms, increasing your inflammation, or keeping you from losing weight (maybe all of these). You may believe this food is healthful for you, but many "health foods" can cause reactions in some people. This is bio-individuality in action.

> One person's food medicine is another person's food problem.

Food Allergies, Intolerances, and Sensitivities: What's the Difference?

Our world has undergone a rapid change over a relatively short period of time. Compared with the total span of human existence, the food we now eat, the water we drink, the depleted soil we grow our crops in, and our polluted environment are all relatively new. Research is looking at this mismatch between our DNA and the world around us as the major driver of chronic inflammatory health problems. Around 99 percent of our genes were formed before the development of agriculture, approximately 10,000 years ago.[1] Because of this mismatch, we are seeing reactions to foods like never before in human history.

Reactions to foods can happen for three primary reasons: allergy, intolerance, or sensitivity. People often conflate, confuse, or misuse these terms, so let's take a look at the differences.

- **Food allergies:** These involve the immune system and have the most immediate and potentially severe response. Symptoms of an allergic reaction can include rashes, itching, hives, swelling, or even anaphylaxis—a swelling of the airways that can be fatal.

The personalized program in this book is *not* for discovering these sorts of life-threatening food reactions. Instead, my aim is to help you discover whether you have either of these two types of food reactivities, which can lead to inflammation:

- **Food intolerances:** Unlike allergies, these do not directly involve the immune system. Instead, intolerances occur when your body is unable to digest certain foods (such as dairy) or when your digestive system becomes irritated by them. These are usually the result of enzyme deficiencies.

- **Food sensitivities:** These are immune-mediated, like allergies, but food sensitivities can result in a more delayed reaction. You might be able to digest a small amount of the food without issues, but overdoing it or eating that food every day could gradually increase your inflammation to the point that your health begins to suffer.

The symptoms of food intolerances and sensitivities include:

- Bloating
- Migraines
- Runny nose
- Brain fog
- Joint or muscle pain
- Anxiety or depression

- Fatigue
- Itching, rashes
- Heart palpitations
- Flu-like symptoms
- Stomachache
- Irritable bowel syndrome

BIO-INDIVIDUALITY AND LIFESTYLE

Bio-individuality is a critical consideration when formulating a dietary strategy, but it applies to more than just food. It applies to almost everything about the way you live your life:

- **Exercise**. Some of my patients flourish on vigorous exercise— for them, it's not only good for their cardiovascular systems but boosts their moods and reduces inflammation. For others, vigorous exercise causes fatigue and stress—for these people, vigorous exercise can be inflammatory, and they do much better with brisk walks in nature, a yoga class, or gentle stretching.

- **Socializing**. One person may get a rush of endorphins from lots of socializing. Social activity may actually be anti-inflammatory for them. Another might feel stressed from too much togetherness in a way that is inflammatory. They will feel best having some alone time.

- **Stress tolerance**. Some people have a high tolerance for stress and even enjoy a fast-paced, challenging day, while others have a low tolerance and need to be more mindful about slowing down, taking time to unplug, and otherwise managing the more stressful aspects of life. We know stress is inflammatory, so it is important to know what stresses *you*.

- **Immunity**. Some people catch every cold, while others hardly ever get run-down. This can be due to the impact of inflammation on your immunity—the more inflamed you are, the more likely you are to get sick.

- **Environment tolerance**. Some people react to every contact with pollution, chemicals, mold, and fungus, while others seem to be immune. Again, for many, these environmental toxins can trigger an inflammatory response, and those who already have more inflammation may also be more sensitive to these toxins.

- **Personality**. Glass half full or half empty? Artistic or logical? We are all different in so many ways, and that too is an aspect of bio-individuality—and related to inflammation.

Bio-individuality is also the main reason a conventional medicine approach helps some people but doesn't help many other people to resolve their symptoms or discover the root of their health or weight issues. This is because doctors who practice conventional medicine are trained in a system oriented toward grouping and categorizing, rather than focusing on the individual.

This is how mainstream medicine diagnoses and treats diseases: When a lot of different people are observed to have the same general set of symptoms and lab test results, their condition is given a name, such as hypothyroidism, rheumatoid arthritis, or depression. These names are given diagnosis codes, which are a set of numbers and letters.

Medications are then assigned to these diagnosis codes based on how well research studies show those medications normalize lab results and diminish symptoms in some percentage of selected groups of people. For example, if medication X relieves the symptoms of fatigue in 52 percent of those whose symptoms match hypothyroidism, then that medication may become a standard prescription for hypothyroidism.

But what about the people whose health issues don't fall into a predetermined set of symptoms? What about the other 48 percent of the people whose symptoms were not relieved by the recommended medication? This medicinal matching game plays the odds, so you can hope that you will be one of the lucky ones, but many people are not. For many, there is no associated medication for their symptoms, so they are sent home without help. For others, the medication assigned doesn't help symptoms because they do not have the same cause as someone else for whom the medication works. Or the medication may relieve the symptoms, but also cause intolerable side effects—sometimes worse than the original symptoms! And then there are those people who question whether they really need to take any drugs. They want to know if there are more natural ways to address their symptoms and a more effective way to stop or reverse the disease process.

Moreover, what if your symptoms are vague and the lab test

results are "normal"? If your symptoms fall neatly into the correct category and the standard medication works to manage your symptoms, great. But if you are an outlier with atypical symptoms or reactions to medications, or if you are more interested in healing your condition than in masking the symptoms with drugs, you may have trouble getting help using this conventional medicine model.

As you can see, there are many exceptions to the rules that define conventional medicine. The patients who represent those exceptions are the ones who most often come to me when the mainstream medical system does not work for them. They are in the group of people who are not helped by the medications they are given, or whose symptoms defy mainstream categorization, or who just aren't getting the help they need.

But the real problem is not that the person's symptoms don't fit some predetermined model. The problem is that the model does not account for bio-individuality. If you gathered five people with the same conventional medicine diagnosis code in a room together, all on the same treatment, and asked each person how his or her treatment was going, you would probably get five different answers because each of those people has different genetics, a different microbiome, and a different biochemistry, and may have quite different reasons for their seemingly similar symptoms. It's a complex picture. Fortunately, it has a common denominator.

THE INFLAMMATION SPECTRUM

Understanding inflammation is one of the most important aspects of understanding how bio-individuality can be used for better health *in you*. When you dive deeply into just about every health problem that we face in the world today—anxiety, depression, fatigue, digestive problems, hormone imbalances, diabetes, heart disease, or autoimmune conditions—they are all inflammatory in nature or have an inflammatory component.

But inflammation is insidious, and it starts brewing in the body long before these diseases become noticeable, not to mention diagnosable. By the time a health problem is advanced enough to be officially diagnosed, inflammation has typically already caused significant damage to the body. For instance, a diagnosis of autoimmune adrenal issues (such as Addison's disease) requires a 90 percent destruction of the adrenal glands.[2] This is true for many other chronic issues—major destruction has to happen for the diagnosis of inflammatory neurological problems like multiple sclerosis or inflammatory gut conditions like celiac disease.

But the inflammation attack that occurs in these conditions does not develop overnight; it's the end-stage event of inflammation. When someone is diagnosed with an autoimmune condition, for example, they have already been experiencing autoimmune inflammation for an average of about four to ten years.[3] The same is true for other chronic inflammatory conditions like diabetes and heart disease. You don't become diabetic overnight. You don't manifest heart disease out of nowhere. Inflammation has been brewing for years before fasting blood sugar is high enough to warrant a diagnosis, or before someone has a heart attack. We all exist somewhere on an inflammation spectrum, from no inflammation to mild to moderate to diagnosis-level inflammation that has resulted in a disease state.

Knowing this, why would anyone wait until they are at the far end of this inflammation spectrum to do something about it? Wouldn't it be much better to take care of inflammation in its earliest stages, when it is much easier to arrest?

The focus of my functional medicine practice is addressing the causes and manifestations of inflammation because the time to start caring about inflammation is long *before* you have a serious health problem. Once you get to the diagnosis stage, the only options typically offered to people are pharmaceutical drugs. I believe we can do much better. My practice and this book are about taking proactive steps to tackle inflammation before it leads to something more serious.

But even if you are already at the point of "serious," there are still many things you can do to reclaim your health. Studies point to what many in functional medicine have been saying for decades: Lifestyle and foods are significant influencers to wellness or a lack of it, and I would add that lifestyle and foods are *the primary methods* for reducing the inflammation that leads to disease. In fact, studies estimate that about 77 percent of inflammatory reactions are determined by factors over which we have at least some control— our diets, our stress levels, and our exposure to pollutants—with the remainder determined by genetics.[4] That means there is much you can do in the here and now to back down the inflammation spectrum rather than moving forward toward chronic disease.

In my experience, the vast majority of us wield quite a bit of power. We can take control of our health in the form of positive lifestyle health interventions right now. Whether those changes improve our quality of life by 25 percent or 100 percent, they're a move in the right direction on the inflammation spectrum. Instead of repeatedly doing the same thing you always have done but expecting different results, you need to try something new. This is the only way to turn negative changes into positive changes.

You are probably reading this book because you have some symptoms you would like to resolve or are struggling with some chronic health issue. Here is a simple fact for you to consider as you mull over bio-individuality and your place on the inflammation spectrum: What *causes inflammation* in you (certain foods, certain exposures, certain kinds of stress) is bio-individual, and what *inflammation causes* in you (weight gain, fatigue, acid reflux) is also bio-individual. However, although inflammation causes a lot of problems, it is also a sort of skeleton key to discovering bio-individual reactions to internal and external stressors. What's great about focusing on inflammation is that:

1. Inflammation is *upstream* from symptoms, meaning that it can cause or worsen many symptoms. Therefore, resolving inflammation can in turn reduce or eliminate the cascade of symptoms downstream that the inflammation caused—multiple symptoms resolved with one attack plan.

2. Inflammation is also downstream from some triggers. A confluence of factors, such as food reactivities, stress, gut problems, infections (bacterial, yeast, or viral), mold or heavy metal toxicities, and genetics is often the driver of inflammation. Cooling inflammation often allows your body to fix the primary dysfunction on its own, resolving the symptoms naturally by eliminating their cause. Inflammation gets in the way of the body's natural ability to heal. If you can discover your own inflammatory triggers (what is causing the inflammation in you) and where your inflammation resides, you can learn how to douse it at its source.

This is how we solve the problem of your health issues: Lower inflammation by customizing your diet and lifestyle to eliminate what is increasing inflammation in you and add what fights inflammation in you. Doing this is likely to directly address your chronic health issues rather than just masking your symptoms.

And how do we customize your diet and lifestyle? We use the information we gain from a personalized and carefully organized elimination diet.

What Exactly Is Inflammation?

Inflammation is your body's natural defense response. In its most acute form, inflammation is the redness, swelling, and pain you get at the site of an injury, such as a scrape, a cut, or a sprained ankle. Inflammation is a product of the immune system. In an inflammatory response, the immune system causes a rush of pro-inflammatory cells to the injury site to keep out bacteria, viruses, and subsequent infection. This is how your body heals. We would all be goners without a healthy, balanced inflammatory response.

The problems start when inflammation gets out of control or out of proportion to the problem, doesn't go away after the injury is healed or the invader is conquered, or when the body activates it mistakenly in response to something that is not actually an invader. When any of these things happen, inflammation becomes its own problem and can trigger many kinds of symptoms in different areas of the body, depending on the cause and site of the inflammation. When inflammation doesn't subside appropriately, continuing for long periods of time at a low level, this is called chronic inflammation. In this state, the immune system can become oversensitive and overreactive, releasing inflammatory cytokines constantly, spreading inflammation system-wide.

In short, when it comes to a healthy inflammation response, it's all about the Goldilocks principle: You don't want too little inflammation, but you don't want too much, either. You want your inflammation to be just right—occurring when necessary, in an amount appropriate for the problem, and then going away when the job is done.

....

An elimination diet will help you discover what foods and behaviors are causing inflammation in you, and where. Because the localization of inflammation into a particular area of the body is bio-individual, influenced by genetics, activities, past injuries, lifestyle choices, and probably other factors we have yet to discover, knowing your inflammation susceptibility and your location on the inflammation spectrum will help you know the best way to improve it. Inflammation tends to develop in eight primary systems:

1. Brain and nervous system

2. Digestive tract

3. Liver, kidneys, and lymphatic system (together, these comprise your body's detoxification system)

4. Liver, pancreas, and cellular insulin receptor sites, which control your blood sugar/insulin balance

5. Endocrine system (the brain's communication with the hormone system: thyroid, adrenals, and ovaries or testes)

6. Muscles, joints, and connective tissue (your musculoskeletal system)

7. Immune system, which can turn against your body, causing autoimmunity

8. Lots of places at once. Some people (many of my patients, in fact) have inflammation in more than one of these areas and/or throughout the body, including in the arteries that go everywhere (which can affect the heart as well as the brain). This may be due either to unusual sensitivity or ignoring inflammation for too long. I refer to this problem as "polyinflammation."

Within each of these areas, inflammation exists on a spectrum, from absent to mild to moderate to extreme—they each have their own inflammation spectrum.

The opposite chart shows you how inflammation in any one area exists on a continuum from mild to extreme, and the different interconnected areas in your body that inflammation can impact. The Inflammation Spectrum Quiz in the next chapter will help you determine your level of inflammation in these different areas and also where you fall on the spectrum for each, so that you can target your problem areas with diet and lifestyle changes.

If you are worried that you might get bad news from this quiz, fear not—no matter where you are on the inflammation spectrum, it is rarely too late to turn things around, and that is exactly what

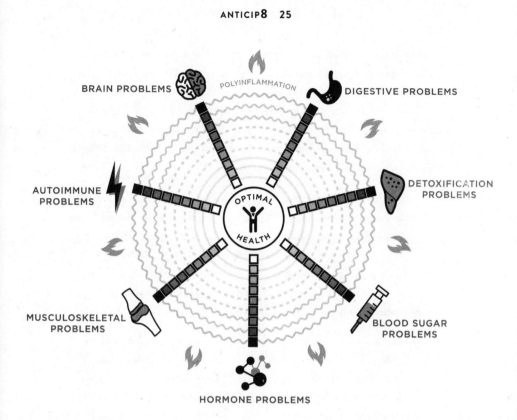

we are going to do. By using an advanced and personalized elimination diet to decrease inflammation triggers in your diet and lifestyle, you will soon learn exactly what you need to do to reverse your direction on the inflammation spectrum.

Inflammation Spectrum Lab Tests

In addition to the quizzes you will take in the next chapter, another way to gauge where your inflammation levels are right now is through testing. Below are some of the lab tests that I run for my patients, to get a comprehensive perspective on where they are on the inflammation spectrum. Although you don't have to get any lab tests to get started tackling inflammation, you could ask your doctor to have some or all these labs run to get a baseline on your inflammation before you start your journey. Having the extra information can motivate you to stay the course and make progress. A functional medicine doctor is likely to be your best source for some of these labs, as this testing is more comprehensive than is standard for conventional medicine. (I run and interpret these labs for people around the world.)

- **hsCRP:** C-reactive protein is an inflammatory protein and this test will show you how much of it you have. The high-sensitivity CRP test is also a surrogate lab to measure IL-6, another pro-inflammatory protein. They are both linked to chronic inflammatory health problems. The optimal range is anything under 1 mg/L. Higher levels are a risk factor for heart disease and can contribute to many other inflammation-based health issues.

- **Homocysteine:** This inflammatory amino acid is linked to heart disease, destruction of the blood-brain barrier, and dementia. It is also commonly elevated in people struggling with autoimmune problems. The optimal range in functional medicine is less than 7 μmol/L.

- **Ferritin:** This lab is normally run to look at stored iron levels, but high levels can also be a sign of inflammation. The optimal range for men is 33–236 ng/mL; premenopausal women: 50–122 ng/mL; postmenopausal women: 150–263 ng/mL.

- **Microbiome labs:** This panel helps assess the health of the gut, where around 80 percent of the immune system resides. By looking at bacterial and yeast overgrowths as well as inflammatory markers like calprotectin and lactoferrin, we can assess gut-centric inflammation.

- **Intestinal permeability:** This blood test looks for antibodies against the proteins that determine the integrity of your gut lining (occludin and zonulin), as well as bacterial toxins called lipopolysaccharides, which can cause inflammation throughout the body.

- **Multiple autoimmune-reactivity labs:** This array shows us if your immune system is creating antibodies against many different parts of the body, such as the brain, thyroid, gut, and adrenal glands. The labs are not meant to diagnose autoimmune disease but rather to look for possible evidence of abnormal autoimmune-inflammation activity.

- **Cross-reactivity labs:** This panel is helpful for gluten-sensitive people who have gone gluten-free and eat a clean diet, but still experience symptoms like digestive problems, fatigue, and neurological symptoms. In these cases, relatively healthy food proteins—such as gluten-free grains, eggs, dairy, chocolate, coffee, soy, and potatoes—may be mistaken by the immune system for gluten, triggering inflammation. To the immune system, it's as if the person never went gluten-free.

- **Methylation gene labs:** Methylation is a biochemical superhighway that regulates many of the functions necessary for a healthy immune system, brain, hormones, and gut. A process occurring about a billion times every second in your body, methylation needs to work well if you are going to work well. Methylation-gene mutations, such as MTHFR, are closely associated with autoimmune inflammation. For example, I have a double mutation at the MTHFR C677t gene; this means that my body is not good at managing an amino acid called homocysteine, which can cause inflammation in some people. I also have autoimmune conditions on both sides of my family, which is a red flag that I need to be even more careful of my place on the inflammation spectrum. You can't change your genes, but by knowing your genetic weaknesses, you can pay extra attention to supporting particular processes in your body to reduce risk factors as much as possible.

- **Cannabinoid Gene CNR1 rs1049353:** Our endocannabinoid system regulates everything from sleep, appetite, pain, inflammation, memory, and mood to reproduction. The cannabinoid gene CNR1 rs1049353 is a significant gene in this system, and changes to this gene are significantly correlated with food sensitivities and autoimmune-inflammation issues. Studies indicate that the gut nervous system is the main site of CB1 cannabinoid receptors.[5]

- APOE4 and APOA2: Variants of these genes affect how the body metabolizes saturated fats. For these gene variants, eating foods higher in saturated fats is associated with inflammatory health problems and weight gain, respectively. People with these gene differences should limit or avoid foods such as dairy, red meat, eggs, coconut products, and other foods higher in saturated fats. Focus instead on plant fats like avocado, olives, and nuts and seeds.

WHAT WILL THIS PROGRAM DO FOR YOU?

The Inflammation Spectrum Quiz in the next chapter will determine your Inflammation Profile, which will illuminate for you the areas that are most reactive in your body and where you fall on the inflammation spectrum. Once you know where you stand, you will follow an elimination diet customized for your specific quiz results, so you can begin proactively decreasing inflammation. If your inflammation is mild, you will do the simplified Core4 track. If it is extreme, or high in multiple areas, you will do the more advanced Elimin8 track. You will also get a toolbox just for your particular area of inflammation, with special medicinal foods, therapies, tips, and tricks to target and attack your inflammation from all angles.

After you follow your prescribed elimination program, your inflammation will be noticeably reduced. At this point you will bring back the foods you eliminated one at time, to see if, in this clear state of reduced inflammation, you still react to them. Then you will finally know what is reactive for you and what is not.

Here's a summary of what you will be doing:

1. Take the Inflammation Spectrum Quiz to determine where you are experiencing inflammation based on your symptoms, where you are on the spectrum of severity in those areas, which area should be your target for intervention with your elimination plan, and which track you will be doing: Core4 or Elimin8.

2. Learn about the Core4 foods that everyone will eliminate (temporarily), and the four additional foods you will eliminate (temporarily) if your quiz results suggest you need a stronger intervention. These are the foods I most often see implicated in inflammation, no matter where it occurs.

3. Get a list of the eight health-damaging lifestyle habits to avoid, and specific information for how to phase them out of your life gradually (and fun things to do instead!).

4. Receive a personalized toolbox for your specific quiz results, which will include safe and therapeutic food medicines to treat your particular areas of inflammation along with targeted therapies—things like herbs, supplements, physical exercises, and lifestyle practices—that I recommend for your set of symptoms and primary area of inflammation.

5. Kick off your plan by eliminating one food item from your list each day, "stepping down" into full elimination diet mode at the end of either four or eight days (depending on whether you do the basic Core4 track or the advanced Elimin8 track).

6. Depending on your quiz score, bask in either four or eight great feel-good weeks of anti-inflammatory living, free from the foods and habits that have been bringing you down. I'll walk you through each week with support, encouragement, fun things to do, delicious meals, and even more ways to support your body as you heal and repair. And don't worry about deprivation or food boredom—you'll have plenty to do and plenty to eat. You'll get easy substitutions for all the things you are giving up, and lots of delectable recipes to enjoy, so anything you might miss will get replaced with something else that will make you feel even better.

7. Enter the Reintegr8 phase by bringing back the foods you eliminated using an organized system of reintroduction. You'll learn how to test each food, in what order, and in what amounts, and how to track any symptom recurrence.

8. Use your Reintegr8 results to create your personalized life list of safe foods to enjoy and foods to leave behind, based on how you have healed and repaired and which foods you now know are nourishing for you and which are still inflammatory. This will allow you to move forward at a new level of health you can continue to build on and maintain, free of dieting dogma and food shame. This is based on what your body—and only your body—has communicated to you through this personalized process.

THE ETHOS BEHIND THIS PROGRAM

When we are talking about eliminating foods for a period of time, it's important to remember why we are doing this in the first place. Eating disorders like orthorexia—obsessive-compulsive anxiety focused on achieving perfection in eating and health habits—are sadly far too common, especially among people going through real health problems who are just trying to find out how to feel better. This program is not about restriction, shame, or self-hate, and it's not an attempt to punish your body by withholding foods. That type of dogmatic dieting consciousness is antithetical to what my work—and this program—is all about. You can't heal a body you hate. Out of self-respect will flow the desire to make healthy choices and the awareness to know what your body needs to thrive. Use this time to bring yourself some calm and bring your body back to center, giving yourself grace, lightness, and forgiveness, maybe for the first time in your life. The heart of *The Inflammation Spectrum* is about loving your body enough to nourish it with delicious, healing foods. It's about caring about yourself enough to find out which foods your body loves and then enjoying those foods. Knowing which foods make you feel terrible and consciously avoiding them isn't punishment—it's an act of self-love.

WHAT'S WITH ALL THE 8S?

In case you haven't noticed, this book is full of the number 8, including the Elimin8 track of the eight-week program for those who fall on the high end of the inflammation spectrum, the eight areas of inflammation, the eight items in every toolbox, the eight chapters and more. Call me a nerd, but I am fascinated by ancient wisdom. One of the things I have learned is the ancient meaning behind 8, which is symbolic of being one step above the natural order and its limitations (7 is a number of completion, and 8 is moving beyond limitations). As I was working on the material for this book, the number 8 kept popping up. It wasn't on purpose at first—I realized there were eight primary ways I commonly see inflammation manifesting in the body. I usually do my elimination diet for at least eight weeks (four for milder cases). There are eight lifestyle habits I typically advise people to kick, and eight chapters I wanted to write. Eight felt right for this book—even spiritual. Eight is about the freedom to move beyond your limitations, and this program is about finding your unique path to that freedom—the indescribable breath of fresh air that happens when we feel and look our best, radiating wellness. Find out what works for your body and what doesn't. This book is your manual to take back your health, once and for all. Are you ready to learn more about how to get *you* back on track and gain food and body peace and freedom for your life by understanding your body better? Let the number 8 be your guide.

2

INVESTIG8: DISCOVER YOUR PERSONALIZED INFLAMMATION PROFILE

Now that you have been thoroughly introduced to bio-individuality and inflammation, it's time to turn the mirror on yourself and figure out where inflammation is rooted in *your* system and where you are on the inflammation spectrum. Do you have uncomfortable symptoms, like weight loss resistance, aching joints, brain fog, skin problems, or mood swings? Do you have digestive problems or irresistible food cravings? Has your doctor told you that you have abnormal labs, like high cholesterol, high blood pressure, or high blood sugar? There is a reason for every negative health issue you are feeling, whether it has ever been diagnosed or not. The key to understanding why you have these symptoms is your *bio-individual inflammation profile*. Functional medicine is also known as *systems medicine*. Which of the eight systems where inflammation can occur is a problem for you? We're going to find out, but let's review the possibilities first. As you read each of these, think about which ones might be relevant in terms of the symptoms and health issues you are experiencing right now:

   1. The brain and nervous system, especially when inflammation has caused a more permeable blood-brain barrier (what is called leaky brain syndrome, similar to leaky gut syndrome) or is causing problems like brain fog, depression, anxiety, trouble concentrating, poor memory, or an overall feeling of unwellness.

2. The digestive tract, including the stomach and the small and large intestines, resulting in digestive problems as well as a "leaky" or more permeable gut lining that can eventually lead to systemic inflammation and even autoimmune disease. Constipation, diarrhea, stomach pain, bloating, and heartburn are just a few of the symptoms.

3. The detoxification system, consisting of the synergistic actions of the liver, kidneys, gallbladder, and lymphatic system. When these are inflamed, they can't process waste as efficiently, meaning it can back up in your system, further exacerbating inflammation, pain, and swelling, such as when your arms, legs, and belly look larger than usual, you have an all-over uncomfortable or painful feeling, or you frequently get rashes.

4. The blood sugar/insulin system, governed by the liver and the pancreas, and cellular insulin receptor sites. When inflammation hits this system, you can experience unstable blood sugar and an excess of insulin, which can eventually lead to metabolic syndrome, prediabetes, or type 2 diabetes. Uncontrolled hunger and thirst as well as sudden rapid weight gain or weight loss resistance are symptoms, as are high fasting blood sugar numbers you might get from a test at your doctor's office.

5. The endocrine system, which consists of the brain's communication with the glands that produce hormones. Inflammation can hit anywhere in this system, impacting the hormones of the thyroid, the adrenal glands, and the sex glands (ovaries or testes), causing a wide range of diverse symptoms—from thinning hair, dry skin, and weak nails to anxiety or mood swings to irregular menstruation or low sex drive—because hormones control so many aspects of wellness.

6. The musculoskeletal or structural system, including muscles, joints, and connective tissue. Inflammation in this system can cause joint pain, muscle pain, joint stiffness, fibromyalgia (a condition often related to autoimmunity), a general feeling of achiness, and more.

7. The immune system, the governing system over inflammation, can overreact and attack the organs, tissues, or structures of the body. This is called autoimmunity. It can happen when inflammation is getting advanced. Autoimmunity can impact every system in the body, especially the digestive system (as with celiac disease or inflammatory bowel disease), the brain and nervous system (as with multiple sclerosis), the joints and connective tissue (as with rheumatoid arthritis and lupus), the thyroid gland (as with Hashimoto's thyroiditis), as well as inflammatory skin conditions.

8. Polyinflammation, which means you have inflammation in more than one area—a common occurrence as inflammation insidiously progresses.

You may already have an idea or two about what your primary areas of inflammation are likely to be, but let's find out in a more objective way. Let's see exactly what areas have been most drastically affected in you in the past few months. This quiz will ask you about your symptoms in each of the above areas. Check all that apply. Afterward, I'll help you score your quiz to determine in which area(s) inflammation is causing the most problems.

THE INFLAMMATION SPECTRUM QUIZ

This quiz will help you determine where inflammation is causing you the most trouble. It's not meant to diagnose you but rather to pinpoint your location on the inflammation spectrum and your area of focus for your elimination plan to determine which track and toolbox is right for you. For each section, answer according to how frequently you have experienced the described condition *in the past one to three months*. If you used to have an issue but don't have it now, don't check that box. Inflammation can migrate, and your old inflammation patterns may have resolved. Once you know your currently active areas of inflammation, your elimination diet plan will help you to tackle them.

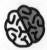

Brain and Nervous System Inflammation Assessment

	NEVER: 0	RARELY: 1	SOMETIMES: 2	OFTEN: 3	ALWAYS: 4
Are you more forgetful than usual—losing things, missing appointments, or forgetting what you are doing or saying?					
Are you depressed for no apparent reason? Have you lost motivation and interest in things you used to enjoy?					
Are you more anxious or worried than usual? Do you get anxiety or panic attacks or feel a general, constant sense of unease or foreboding?					
Do you have "brain fog," or more difficulty concentrating and focusing or staying with one task to completion than usual?					

	NEVER: 0	RARELY: 1	SOMETIMES: 2	OFTEN: 3	ALWAYS: 4
Do you experience unexplained mood swings?					
Do you say words you don't mean to say, or call things by the wrong name, and notice only after you say it or when someone else points it out?					
Do you have sensory issues—i.e., are you experiencing sound, light, or touch in a different way than is normal for you?					
Have you been diagnosed with (or do you suspect you have) mild cognitive decline, and/or do you have a family history of dementia, such as Alzheimer's disease?					

BRAIN AND NERVOUS SYSTEM INFLAMMATION SCORE: _____

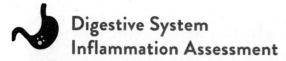

Digestive System Inflammation Assessment

	NEVER: 0	RARELY: 1	SOMETIMES: 2	OFTEN: 3	ALWAYS: 4
Are you often bloated or gassy, and/or does your stomach get distended after or between meals, so that you look pregnant?					
Do you have diarrhea or loose, watery stool that is difficult to control or comes on suddenly?					
Do you get constipated, or go more than twenty-four hours without having a bowel movement, or do you have hard, dry stool that is difficult to pass, resembling small pellets?					
Do you have alternating diarrhea and constipation more often than normal (firm but soft and easy to pass) stools?					

	NEVER: 0	RARELY: 1	SOMETIMES: 2	OFTEN: 3	ALWAYS: 4
Do you get heartburn or acid reflux after eating, when you've gone too long without eating, and/or at night?					
Is your tongue covered with a fuzzy-looking coating, and/or do you have chronic bad breath even when you practice good oral hygiene?					
Does your stomach hurt or cramp, or do you feel sick or nauseated, after eating, whether or not you can associate this with any particular food?					
Do you get uncomfortable stomach or other gastric symptoms (like gas, bloating, or diarrhea) when you are experiencing extreme emotions, such as nervousness, fear, or anxiety?					

DIGESTIVE SYSTEM INFLAMMATION SCORE: _____

Detoxification System Inflammation Assessment

	NEVER: 0	RARELY: 1	SOMETIMES: 2	OFTEN: 3	ALWAYS: 4
Do you retain water easily, and/or feel like your body looks much larger on some days and much smaller and tighter on other days, in a way too extreme or sudden to be related to fat gain or loss? If you press your finger into your lower leg, does it leave a pit for a few seconds?					
Does your weight fluctuate more than five pounds from morning to evening or from one day to the next?					
Have you been diagnosed with any chronic infections such as mold toxicity, Lyme disease, or viral infection?					

	NEVER: 0	RARELY: 1	SOMETIMES: 2	OFTEN: 3	ALWAYS: 4
Do you have a vague feeling of "being toxic," even if you can't pin it on any particular symptom?					
Have you noticed a yellowish tint to your skin or the whites of your eyes?					
Do you have abdominal tenderness that seems unrelated to eating, especially in the upper right quadrant of your torso, or that spreads to your upper back or shoulder?					
Does your urine tend to be dark yellow, and/or does your stool tend to float?					
Do you have unexplained itching, flaking, or rashes on your hands and/or feet?					

DETOXIFICATION SYSTEM INFLAMMATION SCORE: _____

Blood Sugar/Insulin System Inflammation Assessment

	NEVER: 0	RARELY: 1	SOMETIMES: 2	OFTEN: 3	ALWAYS: 4
Do you crave sugary or starchy foods even when you have already eaten enough or feel full (such as after a big meal or too soon between meals)?					
Have you noticed an increase in appetite and/or thirst and urination recently?					
Do you get blurred vision that comes and goes?					
Are you unusually tired even if you got enough sleep but notice that your fatigue is relieved by eating something?					

	NEVER: 0	RARELY: 1	SOMETIMES: 2	OFTEN: 3	ALWAYS: 4
Do you feel light-headed, dizzy, shaky, jittery, irritable, or "hangry" (a combination of hungry and angry) when you haven't eaten for a few hours or you skip a meal?					
Is your waist girth equal to or greater than your hip girth?					
Do you have difficulty losing weight, even when cutting calories and/or exercising?					
Have you had your fasting blood sugar tested and it was 100 dl/ml or higher, and/or have you had a hemoglobin A1C test and it was 5.7 or above, and/or do you have a diagnosis of prediabetes, metabolic syndrome, or type 2 diabetes?					

BLOOD SUGAR/INSULIN SYSTEM

INFLAMMATION SCORE: _____

Hormonal (Endocrine) System Inflammation Assessment

	NEVER: 0	RARELY: 1	SOMETIMES: 2	OFTEN: 3	ALWAYS: 4
Do you tend to have fatigue and/or headaches in the afternoons, then get a second wind in the evening, which causes you to stay up late?					
Do you feel dizzy when you stand up suddenly?					
Do you often crave salty foods?					
Are your hands and feet often cold, even when your environment is warm?					
Do you sleep excessively, or feel as if you could sleep all day and still sleep at night?					
Are the outer thirds of your eyebrows thinning or missing?					

	NEVER: 0	RARELY: 1	SOMETIMES: 2	OFTEN: 3	ALWAYS: 4
Has your sex drive disappeared? Are you rarely if ever "in the mood"?					
For women: Are you experiencing irregular, painful, or unusually heavy menstrual periods? **For men:** Have you recently experienced any new occurrence of erectile dysfunction?					

HORMONAL (ENDOCRINE) SYSTEM INFLAMMATION SCORE: _____

Musculoskeletal System Inflammation Assessment

	NEVER: 0	RARELY: 1	SOMETIMES: 2	OFTEN: 3	ALWAYS: 4
Do your joints hurt periodically, constantly, or in flares, in random places, with the pain coming and going, seemingly unrelated to injuries?					
Are you hypermobile, "double-jointed," or are your joints hyper-flexible?					
Are you accident-prone, often twisting your ankle, tripping or falling, or dropping things? Do you consider yourself clumsy? Do you often injure your tendons and/or ligaments?					
Do your joints constantly pop, crack, snap, or get stuck in certain positions?					

	NEVER: 0	RARELY: 1	SOMETIMES: 2	OFTEN: 3	ALWAYS: 4
Do you wake up with stiff and/or aching joints and/or muscles but can relieve the stiffness by movement, only to find that it returns at the end of an active day?					
Do you have chronic neck or back pain, tightness, and tension?					
Do you get pins and needles, random stabbing pains, and/or numbness in your hands and feet, or shooting pains down your arms or legs?					
Are massages painful, especially in your arms, legs, and buttocks?					

MUSCULOSKELETAL SYSTEM INFLAMMATION SCORE: _____

Autoimmune-Inflammation Assessment

	NEVER: 0	RARELY: 1	SOMETIMES: 2	OFTEN: 3	ALWAYS: 4
Are you experiencing obvious extreme reactions to certain foods or after eating—reactions such as vomiting, diarrhea, pain, skin reactions, or neurological episodes like brain fog or panic attacks?					
Are you intolerant to cold or heat, and/or do your hands or feet turn bluish or gray when they are cold? And/or are your skin, mouth, or eyes unusually dry?					
Do you have a family history of autoimmune issues, such as rheumatoid arthritis, lupus, multiple sclerosis, celiac disease, inflammatory bowel disease/Crohn's disease, or Hashimoto's thyroiditis?					
Do you have joint pain and swelling, and/or numbness and tingling, bilaterally (in the same place on both sides of your body, such as in both hands, elbows, knees, and/or feet)?					

	NEVER: 0	RARELY: 1	SOMETIMES: 2	OFTEN: 3	ALWAYS: 4
Do you have unexplained rashes, chronic acne, or recurring boils or cystic acne on your face or body?					
Do you have extreme, constant, unrelenting fatigue that cannot be relieved by sleeping, eating, or other remedies?					
Are you having unexplained muscle weakness, or have you noticed that your foot is dragging or you are dropping things more often?					
Are any of the above symptoms episodic, flaring up, sometimes to an extreme degree, then dying down for a while, only to return days, weeks, or even months later?					

AUTOIMMUNE-INFLAMMATION SCORE:_____

To determine your total quiz score, add up all your scores. Write that number here. You will need to refer to it shortly:

YOUR TOTAL QUIZ SCORE: _____

 Polyinflammation Assessment

We'll handle this category a bit differently because it is not its own inflammation system but a collection of the above systems. Look back over your quiz answers and check any of the categories in which you scored eight points or more:

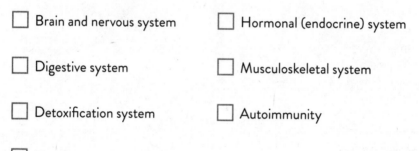

☐ Brain and nervous system   ☐ Hormonal (endocrine) system

☐ Digestive system   ☐ Musculoskeletal system

☐ Detoxification system   ☐ Autoimmunity

☐ Blood sugar/insulin system

If you checked more than one of these boxes, you should consider yourself in the Polyinflammation category. Don't worry—many of my patients fall into this category. It means inflammation is more widespread in your system, but that is all the more reason to take action now, before it gets any worse!

Scoring

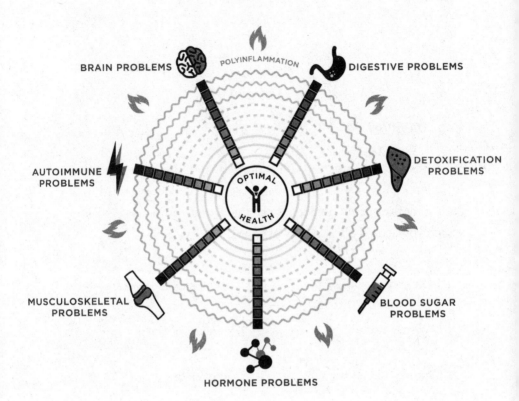

The next step is to determine what your quiz is telling you about where inflammation is most aggravating your system, and how severe it is—in other words, where you fall on the Inflammation Spectrum. Your score will determine which level of the program you will do: the Core4 track or the Elimin8 track. It will also direct you to your appropriate personalized toolbox.

You should have seven scores, one for each inflammation-prone area; either a yes or a no regarding your qualification for the Polyinflammation category; and a total quiz score, which is the combined totals of the seven other scores. For easy reference, copy them here:

....

QUIZ SCORE SUMMARY

BRAIN AND NERVOUS SYSTEM INFLAMMATION SCORE _____

DIGESTIVE SYSTEM INFLAMMATION SCORE _____

DETOXIFICATION SYSTEM INFLAMMATION SCORE _____

BLOOD SUGAR/INSULIN SYSTEM INFLAMMATION SCORE _____

HORMONAL (ENDOCRINE) SYSTEM INFLAMMATION SCORE _____

MUSCULOSKELETAL SYSTEM INFLAMMATION SCORE _____

AUTOIMMUNE-INFLAMMATION SCORE _____

POLYINFLAMMATION: Did you score 8 or more points in more than one category above? Yes/No

YOUR TOTAL QUIZ SCORE _____

....

Each separate system on the inflammation spectrum exists on a continuum from mild to severe inflammation. Here is what your scores in each individual system mean:

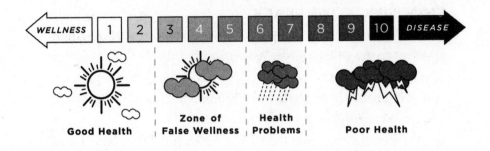

Zero to 2: Congratulations! You are pretty much inflammation free in this particular area and may not need to focus on this system for now.

Between 3 and 5: You have some inflammation in this area, but your symptoms are probably not significant or obvious yet and are likely not impacting your life too much. But watch out—I call this the Zone of False Wellness, when people feel pretty good most of the time, never suspecting an inflammation storm is brewing. If you don't address inflammation in your most severe areas, these "false wellness" zones may soon join the (very unfun) party and your health will decline.

Between 6 and 7: Inflammation is progressing here, not yet severe but enough to get your full attention. However, this area deserves your attention because the inflammation storm is definitely developing and starting to rile up your system and show some symptoms.

8 or higher: Areas with scores of 8 or above are the areas in which inflammation has progressed significantly. These should be your most immediate areas of concern.

CHOOSING YOUR TRACK

There are various ways to choose which track of the elimination plan you will do. Here is how to decide:

DO THE CORE4 TRACK IF:

- You have only one system with a score of 8 or more.

- Your total quiz score is 15 or less.

- You just want to lean into this process in a way that is easier and that you feel is doable for you at this point in your life.

DO THE ELIMIN8 TRACK IF:

- You scored 8 or higher in two or more systems (i.e., your bio-individual inflammation profile is Polyinflammation).

- Your total quiz score is 16 or higher.

- You want to "go big or go home" and you feel ready to tackle your inflammation as much as you can right now.

Let's summarize your results:

1. Your **bio-individual inflammation profile** is the area where you scored the highest. This will determine which toolbox you get. Record the result below, and if two or more areas are tied, list them all.

2. Your **track** is the plan you will be doing, either Core4 or Elimin8. This will determine your food list and meal plan options. Record your result below.

....

My bio-individual inflammation profile—area(s) of most concern—is:

_____

My track is (circle one): Core4/Elimin8

....

Finally, I would like you to list your eight worst symptoms. You will refer back to this list later, to monitor your progress. You may have more than eight symptoms, but choose the eight that most severely impact your life, health, function, or happiness right now. What bothers you the most in your life right now? Headaches? Constipation? Joint pain? Heartburn? Low energy? Anxiety? Weight loss resistance? An abnormal test result? Or something else? If you have fewer than eight, great! Just list the ones you most want to resolve.

My Eight Worst Symptoms Right Now

1._____

2._____

3._____

4._____

5._____

6._____

7._____

8._____

Now you know your profile and your track, you have symptom relief goals, and you understand bio-individuality. Awesome! Everything from here on out will be about exactly what you are going to do to get your health and life back under your control. The first thing we're going to do is give you a personalized toolbox so that you have what you need to take action.

3

INCORPOR8: YOUR TRACK AND YOUR TOOLBOX

Now it's time to find out exactly what you will be doing on your particular track of the elimination phase, whether it's the Core4 track or the Elimin8 track, and to get your personalized toolbox, which will contain extra therapies, like special foods to focus on, supplements to take, and practices that all address your bio-individual inflammation profile. In the next chapter, I will go into more detail about why you will be doing what you are doing, but right now let's get to the nuts and bolts.

IF YOU ARE DOING THE CORE4 TRACK

First, let's look at what you will be doing if you have chosen to do the Core4 track, based on your quiz results from the previous chapter.

Welcome to Your Core4 Track

If you have decided to do the Core4 track, your basic plan will look like this:

1. You will be eliminating four primary foods that are most likely to be inflammatory. To do this, you will step down over four days, eliminating one inflammatory food each day, to adjust gradually to a new way of eating.

2. Next you will spend four weeks living without those foods, trying new foods, living an anti-inflammatory lifestyle, and choosing and eliminating four (or more) inflammatory habits I will tell you about, based on what you believe is most problematic for you.

3. After four weeks, you will reintroduce the four foods you have eliminated, one at a time, through a specific and organized method, to determine which of these foods are inflammatory for you. After calming down your system and your inflammation, you will be able to perceive genuine reactions to your personal inflammatory foods.

4. Finally, based on what you learned from the elimination diet program, you will create a personalized life list of foods that are good for you, and foods to avoid, for a lifetime of anti-inflammatory health-building and thriving.

The Core4 Foods to Eliminate

These are the four food categories you will be eliminating gradually during your four-day step-down and completely during the four-week inflammation-cooling phase. These are the foods that are mostly likely to cause inflammation in most people:

1. Grains. You will be eliminating all grains (even those without gluten). Many people have an inflammatory reaction to grains of all types, and this is the only way we can determine whether you are one of those people. That means crossing off wheat, rye, barley, rice, corn, oats, spelt, quinoa, and anything made with them from your list of available foods for now.

2. Dairy products containing lactose and casein, including animal-derived milk, yogurt, ice cream, cheese, and coffee creamer. These foods are also common sources of inflammation. Although you may do okay with dairy products, you won't know for sure until you eliminate them for a while.

3. Added sweeteners of all types, especially cane sugar, corn syrup, and agave syrup, but also maple syrup, honey, date syrup, coconut sugar, stevia, monk fruit, sugar alcohols like xylitol, and anything else you add to foods to make them sweeter than they are naturally. While the more processed sweeteners are more likely to cause inflammation in most people, you may find, when testing during reintroduction, that you can bring some natural sugars back into your diet. Or you may find that added sweeteners don't agree with you at all. In order for you to find out for sure, they are all eliminated for now.

4. Inflammatory oils, especially corn, soy, canola, sunflower, grape-seed, and vegetable oils, as well as trans fats (anything that says "partially hydrogenated"). These guys are highly processed and likely to be inflammatory for you. The real test will be taking them out of your diet, then reintroducing them later.

IF YOU ARE DOING THE ELIMIN8 TRACK

Now let's look at what you will be doing if you have chosen to do the Elimin8 track, based on your quiz results from the previous chapter. Here is your plan:

Welcome to Your Elimin8 Track

If you are one of those rock stars who chooses the Elimin8 track (either because of your quiz results or just because you like to go hard or go home), this is how your plan will look:

1. You will eliminate eight inflammatory foods, including the Core4 foods listed above, plus four additional foods that are commonly inflammatory for many people. This is a stronger intervention into your inflammation. You will step down over eight days, eliminating one inflammatory food each day, to adjust to this new way of eating.

2. Next, you will spend eight weeks living without those eight foods, trying new anti-inflammatory foods, living an anti-inflammatory lifestyle, and eliminating up to eight possible inflammatory habits you have chosen from the list I will give you, that you feel are most problematic for you.

3. After eight weeks, you will reintroduce the eight foods you have eliminated one at a time, through a specific and organized method, to determine which of these foods are inflammatory for you. Because you have cooled your inflammation, your system will be sensitized to these foods that have been out of your life. If you are truly intolerant of them, you will know it!

4. Finally, you will create a personalized life list of foods that are good for you, and foods to avoid, for a lifetime of anti-inflammatory health-building and thriving.

The Elimin8 Foods to Eliminate

You will be eliminating the same foods as those on the Core4 Track, so read about those on pages 57–58. You will also be eliminating four additional foods, so you can *slay* that inflammation and get back on the road to optimal health. Here are your eight potentially inflammatory no-gos for now (until reintroduction):

1. **Grains**

2. **Dairy products**

3. **Added sweeteners**

4. **Inflammatory oils**

5. **Legumes**, such as lentils, black beans, pinto beans, white beans, peanuts, and anything made from soy. These contain lectins,

phytates, and other potentially inflammatory proteins.[1] Some people do fine with legumes, but many don't. You will find out where you stand during reintroduction.

6. Nuts and seeds, including almonds, cashews, hazelnuts, walnuts, sunflower seeds, pumpkin seeds, and sesame seeds. For some people, these are hard to digest (especially if they are not soaked beforehand) and contain many of the same potentially inflammatory compounds as legumes.

7. Eggs, both whole eggs and egg whites. My body loves eggs (and so do I), but many people are sensitive to the albumin in egg whites, and some are sensitive to the whole egg. We'll find out if you are one of them.

8. Nightshades, including tomatoes, tomatillos, sweet and hot peppers, white potatoes, eggplant, and goji berries. These contain alkaloids that are more inflammatory for some people. Maybe you.

....

About Caffeine and Alcohol

You may be surprised that caffeine and alcohol are not part of the Core4 or Elimin8 lists. Actually, I do want you to eliminate these, but I don't add them to the list because they aren't actual foods. However, both can be inflammatory in multiple ways. Primarily, caffeine can stress your brain-adrenal communication and alcohol is an added burden on your liver. Since the goal is to bring down inflammation in both these areas, caffeine and alcohol are best left out. But don't worry—I'm not telling you that you have to go for the rest of your life without a glass of wine or a nice hot cup of coffee. During the Reintegr8 phase, you can test them to see if you react to them. The only way to know, however, is to get them out of your system for a while first.

There is one and only one exception. I give you the thumbs-up to enjoy one to four cups of organic green or white tea each day. These inflammation-lowering drinks are lower in caffeine and can also be useful if you are used to drinking a lot of caffeinated beverages (hello, coffee) because they can ease the caffeine withdrawal headache.

....

A SPECIAL NOTE FOR VEGETARIANS AND VEGANS

I have had many patients over the years come to me who were vegetarian or vegan, and as I wrote about at length in *Ketotarian*, I, myself, was a vegan for ten years, so I understand the deeply rooted motivations for this lifestyle. I respect it, I have lived it, and I would never tell you to cast aside your personal beliefs, nor would I discount your legitimate point of view. That being said, I also want you to understand that while you are on this elimination phase, if you also eliminate all sources of animal protein, you may discover that there is limited food left to eat. While I am a huge fan of being plant-centric, many categories of plant foods that vegetarians and vegans typically eat a lot of (like grains, legumes, nuts, seeds, and nightshades) can be inflammatory for some people. Since our goal is to reduce inflammation significantly so that we can determine which foods cause inflammation in *you*, this may require a bit of a reframing. But let's talk about it, because it's not a deal-breaker.

In my experience, people avoid meat or all animal products for religious, ethical, or health reasons. They also have varying commitments to the lifestyle. First, let me address all of you who are vegetarian or vegan right now but think you might be willing to consider a different diet, at least temporarily, if it could help you with your health goals.

If You Are Flexible

Many of my vegetarian or vegan patients have come to me at a point in their lives when they were desperate to feel better and were willing to entertain the idea that their diets were not best for their bodies. There is nothing wrong with vegetarian or vegan diets if they are working for you. These diets work great for many people, but because of bio-individuality they do not work great for everyone.

The people who come to me are not among those who are thriving. They don't feel good, and the best way to make a change is with diet. If you want to feel different, you must do something different. Many vegetarians get most of their protein from eggs and dairy products, which could be potentially inflammatory for them. Vegans especially tend to eat a large amount of high-carbohydrate foods containing lectins and phytates (grains, nuts, seeds, and legumes), which are potentially inflammatory anti-nutrients. You can't live on air and ice cubes, so if you choose to try eliminating many of the most inflammatory foods to calm your inflammation and get ahead of your health issues, you have only so many foods left to choose from. That could mean that you may need to bring back some animal products (while still being plant-centric), at least for a while.

> **If you want to feel different, you must do something different.**

The purpose of this individualized elimination program is to assess, objectively, what works best for your body. But this is just an experiment. It isn't forever. You might discover that a vegetarian or vegan diet serves you just fine, once you isolate those particular foods that cause inflammation in you and eliminate those. Or you might discover that your body does much better on completely different foods than you have been eating. Unless you are willing to be flexible about what you eliminate, it will be much more difficult to nail down exactly which foods and behaviors are problematic for you. Also, if your list of allowable foods becomes so short that it can't provide you with adequate nutrition, you won't get good results because you won't be giving your body what it needs to heal and flourish.

I encourage you to try some animal protein and see what happens—even if it's just some fish and/or seafood, while still being mostly plant-based. I have no judgment or agenda, other than a desire to see you discover more about your bio-individuality and resolve your health issues. You don't have to have it at every meal. Ease in if you can, and during reintroduction you will see how you feel on the other vegan and vegetarian staples you removed during the elimination phase.

If Animal Protein Is a No-Way, No-How Proposition for You

For those of you who are absolutely 100 percent opposed to eating any animal products now and forever, I completely understand and empathize with that. There are ways to work around your restrictions. Your results may not be as clear or effective, but you will likely still discover valuable information about your own reactivities. If this is you, modify your plan like this:

1. Just do the Core4 track for now, even if your quiz results suggest that you should do the Elimin8 track. See how you respond to it. This will start to calm inflammation down, while still allowing for legumes, fermented soy like tempeh and natto, nuts and seeds, and (if you eat them) eggs. It will still make a difference.

2. Or do the Elimin8 track, but make an exception for small amounts of legumes, nuts, and seeds.

3. When you eat legumes, nuts, and seeds, always soak them in purified water for at least eight hours before cooking and eating them (or before drying them in a dehydrator, in the case of nuts and seeds), for maximum reduction of potentially inflammatory elements (lectins and phytates). Cooking beans and other legumes such as lentils in a pressure cooker is also an option, as this is quicker and will also reduce the potentially inflammatory lectin and phytic acid content of these foods.

4. No matter which plan you choose, eat as many green vegetables as possible every single day. This is a powerful way to bring down inflammation.

5. Focus on low-fructose fruit, to keep your blood sugar more stable in the absence of animal protein. See the complete list on page 114.

6. For a good protein source, use organic non-GMO fermented-only soy like tempeh or natto, or try hempfu, which is like tofu but made with hempseed. (Avoid processed soy products like packaged veggie "burgers" and veggie "hot dogs," as well as unfermented soy products like tofu and soy milk. Organic edamame is permitted.

7. Choose plenty of healthy plant fats, such as coconuts, avocados, and olives (and their oils); coconut milk and yogurt (unsweetened); and almond milk and yogurt (unsweetened).

8. You might discover upon reintroduction that some grains work for you, but keep them off your list for now. The same for dairy, if you normally eat it. All the Core4 food items still apply to you during the elimination phase, no exceptions.

If you still aren't feeling better after four weeks:

- Look at your protein sources. If you have been eating soy, are you eating only organic, non-GMO fermented soy foods (such as tempeh and natto)? If not, be stricter about this, or eliminate all soy foods. You may be reacting to them.

- If you are eating eggs, consider eliminating the whites, which tend to be the most inflammatory part, due to their albumin content. Or eliminate whole eggs, in case you are more sensitive.

- If you are eating a lot of nuts and seeds, are you soaking them first? Be sure to do this every time. If you are soaking them, try going without nuts and seeds for a few days to see if you notice a change.

- Maybe you have been eating too many legumes or you are reactive to a particular legume. Give yourself a legume break every few days. Instead, make soups a few evenings in a row, full of a wide variety of mushrooms, ginger and/or galangal, and lots of fresh herbs, spices, and vegetables, pureed if you are having digestive issues.

- You could also try isolating different legumes to see if you do better on some than on others. Don't forget to soak them first! Presoaked or pressure-cooked lentils and mung beans tend to be less reactive than other legumes like black beans or pinto beans.

BIO-INDIVIDUAL TOOLBOXES

Your bio-individual inflammation profile (which you wrote down on page 53) determines your assigned toolbox, so find the one that matches your most pressing issue (according to your quiz results) and dip into it for extra anti-inflammatory power. Keep it handy by making a copy or bookmarking the page where your toolbox starts so you can refer to it often. The bonus therapies in these toolboxes are optional, but they will definitely boost the effectiveness of your inflammation-dampening efforts. All of the supplement and food medicines in the toolboxes can be found in most health food stores or online. I suggest looking at your local health food store and talking with the staff for the best brands they have in stock or reading customer reviews online. New brands come onto the market all the time, so this is the best way to vet which one to try.

Brain/Nervous System Toolbox

Is your brain on fire? Is your nervous system aflame? Signs of brain inflammation include brain fog, problems with concentration and focus, mood problems like anxiety and/or depression, and memory issues. Long-term brain inflammation may be a risk factor for cognitive impairment and eventually dementia, as well as for autoimmune disease or other neurological conditions like Parkinson's, especially in genetically susceptible people. A leaky blood-brain barrier could be to blame. This is a condition often linked to leaky gut syndrome, and it means that the tight junctions that seal off the digestive system and the brain have become compromised. This can let bacterial endotoxins, called lipopolysaccharides (LPS), into places they shouldn't be, triggering an inflammatory response.

Your toolbox contains the foods and other therapies that target brain inflammation. You will probably notice an improvement in your mood and ability to concentrate within just a few days of beginning this plan. Here are your tools. Eat them, use them, try them, as often as you can.

1. Wild-caught fish, because of its high concentration of brain-boosting docosahexaenoic acid (DHA), an omega-3 fatty acid.[2]

2. MCT oil: its bioavailable fats, extracted from coconut and palm oil, have been shown to improve cognitive function.[3]

3. Lion's mane mushroom, which contains nerve growth factors (NGFs) to help regenerate and protect brain tissue.[4]

4. *Mucuna pruriens*, an Ayurvedic herb that supports the central and peripheral nervous systems, helping the body to adapt to stress. It is rich in L-dopa, the precursor to the neurotransmitter dopamine.[5][6] It is sometimes called *kapikacchu*.

5. Krill oil is even better than fish oil, containing 50 times more of the powerful antioxidant astaxanthin than most fish oil brands. Krill oil also contains the beneficial phospholipids called phosphatidylcholine and phosphatidylserine, which the body uses to support brain and nerve function.[7] [8]

6. Magnesium supports the brain receptors for learning and memory function, increasing neuroplasticity and mental clarity.[9] [10] Deficiencies have been linked to brain problems such as anxiety, depression, ADHD, migraines, and brain fog. Magnesium glycinate and magnesium threonate are two of the most absorbable forms that are conducive to calming anxiety and improving cognitive function (respectively).

7. Aerobic exercise enhances the production of BDNF (brain-derived neurotrophic factor), boosting memory and overall cognitive function.[11] [12] Try to get at least 30 minutes six days per week.

8. Valerian root, which contains valerenic acid, a substance that modulates the neurotransmitter GABA.[13] Brain-derived neurotrophic factor (BDNF) is a protein that helps the growth and function of neurons.[14] Healthy GABA levels are necessary for increasing BDNF,[15] which is important because low BDNF levels are associated with impaired memory and Alzheimer's.[16]

Mantra: *My thoughts are aligned with perfect health, and I become clearer and happier each day.*

Repeat this mantra aloud or in your mind whenever you think of it throughout the day, and for 5 to 15 minutes while sitting quietly in the morning and/or evening. This is a form of meditation.

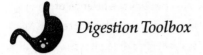 *Digestion Toolbox*

I find that almost everyone experiencing chronic health issues has some degree of gut inflammation resulting in digestive dysfunction, even if it's mild. The most common issues I see in my clinic are constipation, diarrhea, irritable bowel syndrome (IBS), small intestinal bacterial overgrowth (SIBO), bloating, and acid reflux. Chronic digestive issues can also cause other serious problems, such as esophageal damage from long-term acid reflux, or a stomach or intestinal ulcer, as well as loosening the junctions in the gut lining, causing leaky gut syndrome, which can trigger autoimmune problems. Calming inflammation in your digestive tract so it can heal and work better can have a ripple effect throughout your entire system. Make this happen now with your toolbox. Here are your tools to try—use them often.

1. **Cooked vegetables** instead of raw. They are much easier to digest. Pureeing them in a blender for soup or to add to other foods makes them even more digestible.

2. **Bone broth and galangal broth.** Cook bone broth (page 252) no more than eight hours or pressure-cook it to reduce the effect of inflammatory histamines that develop with extended cooking times. Galangal broth (page 253), made from galangal, a root related to ginger, is a plant-based option. Both are anti-inflammatory, healing for the gut, and can be sipped by themselves or used as a base for soups. Try them both, if you can. They are easy to make.

3. **Fermented vegetables and drinks.** Vegetables like sauerkraut and kimchi and drinks such as water or coconut kefir, beet kvass, and kombucha contain beneficial bacteria to restore and support good gut bacteria.[17] (Avoid sweetened versions of fermented drinks.)

4. Probiotic supplements. These help improve the balance of bacteria in your gut. Rotate different ones for greater bacterial diversity.[18] [19]

5. L-glutamine supplements. This amino acid supports healing of the gut lining.[20] [21]

6. Digestive enzymes such as betaine HCL with pepsin and ox bile. These enzymes can support your body's digestion of protein and fat as your gut heals.

7. Deglycyrrhizinated licorice supplement. Licorice root is soothing and healing for an inflamed gut lining.

8. Slippery elm powder. This is an excellent remedy for irritable bowel syndrome issues like cramping, bloating, and gas.[22] It's also healing for the gut lining.

Mantra: *I am in perfect balance and I trust my gut.*

Repeat this mantra aloud or in your mind throughout the day, and for 5 to 15 minutes while sitting quietly in the morning and/or evening. This mantra works well for digestive issues because trusting your gut means you trust it to heal, but you also trust your own intuition—your "gut feeling."

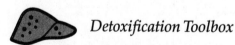 *Detoxification Toolbox*

Your liver, lymphatic system, kidneys, and gallbladder are largely responsible for detoxification as well as processing and removing toxins like alcohol and drugs, pesticides and pollutants, and the waste products of your own metabolism. If these systems get impaired by inflammation, waste can back up in your body, causing more inflammation. If your quiz suggests that you are having inflammatory issues with your detoxification system, you could be prone to lymphatic backup, fatty liver disease, gallbladder problems, or a feeling of being "toxic." You might also be letting toxins hang around in your body too long, where they can cause damage to organs and systems. This category also encompasses those who may be struggling with Lyme disease, mold exposure, or heavy alcohol or drug use, or who have to take prescription drugs every day. Cool the inflammation in your detox system ASAP with the liver/lymphatic/gallbladder toolbox and free up your body's natural systems for taking out the trash. Here is your toolbox.

1. Dandelion tea. A natural liver tonic, this tea contains B vitamins to support methylation and detoxification.[23]

2. Spirulina supplements or powder. This alga has potent detoxification properties.[24]

3. Red clover blossom tea, powder, or supplements. This is another liver supporter that helps promote efficient detoxification.

4. Milk thistle tea or supplements. Yet another liver supporter that can help decrease heavy metal damage.[25] [26]

5. Parsley and cilantro, which help eliminate heavy metals such as lead and mercury. Add these herbs, fresh or dried, to your meals.

6. Sulfur-containing vegetables. Vegetables with a high sulfur content include garlic, onions, Brussels sprouts, cabbage, cauliflower, broccoli, and broccoli sprouts. These help your liver break down toxins and heavy metals, making it easier for your body to get rid of them. Broccoli sprouts are even more powerful than broccoli. Their sulforaphane content aids in supporting healthy detoxification pathways. Try to have some of these vegetables every day.

7. Leafy greens. Dark leafy greens like kale, spinach, and chard contain folate, which is essential for opening detox pathways. Bitter greens, such as collard greens, mustard greens, and arugula, also support liver function.

8. Dry brushing. Special dry brushes are made for brushing your skin before showering. Brush up legs and arms toward the body, and brush the torso toward the armpits and groin, or toward the center of the body, where you have the highest concentration of lymph nodes. Dry brushing daily gets your lymphatic system working and moves excess fluid and lymph out of the body, along with the waste they carry. This can eliminate that puffy look, which comes from sluggish lymph. Do it right before you take a shower or bath.

Mantra: *I allow my body to return to its most natural state of thriving health. I am cleansed and pure.*

Repeat this mantra aloud or in your mind whenever you think of it, and for 5 to 15 minutes while sitting quietly in the morning and/or evening. It will help you cleanse body, mind, and spirit.

 Blood Sugar/Insulin Toolbox

If your blood sugar goes too high too often, you are at risk for insulin resistance in all its various forms: metabolic syndrome, prediabetes, obesity, and eventually full-blown type 2 diabetes, including its many complications (nerve pain, cardiovascular disease, kidney damage, and vision damage, to name a few). Diabetes is no joke, taking an average of ten years off a life. Some experts believe half of all U.S. citizens have some degree of insulin resistance. Contributors to this imbalance may be inflammation in the liver and exhausted cellular insulin receptors in the liver that are no longer sensitive to insulin's sugar-balancing effects. Diet is essential in managing blood sugar and insulin balance, to reduce liver inflammation and modify extreme changes in blood sugar and insulin that can result in diabetes. If your quiz results suggest you have a problem with this, it's time to get off the blood sugar roller coaster and jump right on the blood sugar/insulin plan. This is your toolbox.

1. Cinnamon. Try cinnamon tea, or add cinnamon to your warm drinks, fruit, or other food. This tree bark contains proanthocyanidins, which alter insulin-signaling activity in fat cells in a positive way. Cinnamon has been shown to reduce blood sugar levels and triglycerides in people with type 2 diabetes.[27]

2. Reishi mushrooms. Most available as a tea, powder, or dried, these medicinal mushrooms help lower blood sugar levels by downregulating alpha-glucosidase, the enzyme responsible for breaking down starches into sugars.[28]

3. Berberine supplements. Berberine is a plant-based alkaloid and a remedy in Chinese medicine that delays the breakdown of carbohydrates into sugars,[29] keeps blood sugar levels balanced, and has been shown to be just as effective as metformin[30] in regulating blood sugar in people with diabetes.

4. Matcha. This form of green tea contains a compound called epigallocatechin-3-gallate (EGCG), which helps stabilize blood sugar.[31] Drinking the whole green tea leaf in the form of matcha powder is a great way to increase your intake of EGCG.

5. D-chiro-inositol supplements. This nutrient plays an important role in insulin signaling and decreases insulin resistance.[32]

6. Apple cider vinegar. This common kitchen ingredient greatly improves insulin sensitivity and improves the way your body responds to sugar[33] in addition to encouraging lower fasting blood sugar levels.[34]

7. High-fiber vegetables. Fiber from whole-food plant sources is particularly effective at both improving insulin sensitivity and lowering glucose metabolism.[35]

8. Chromium supplements. Chromium is a mineral that plays a role in insulin-signaling pathways. It improves insulin sensitivity and blood glucose in addition to lowering triglyceride and cholesterol levels.[36]

Mantra: *My blood sugar is balanced, I am balanced. My insulin and leptin hormones are balanced, I am balanced.*

Repeat this mantra aloud or in your mind randomly throughout the day, and for 5 to 15 minutes while sitting quietly in the morning and/or evening. This calming activity centered on balance can have a positive mind-body influence. Stress can trigger higher blood sugar levels, so the stress-reversing action of this mantra will enhance your efforts.

 Hormone (Endocrine System) Toolbox

If you suffer from moodiness, PMS, irregular or painful periods, or a low sex drive, or you are heading toward menopause and having a lot of uncomfortable symptoms, you probably already suspect that you are having trouble with your hormone balance. These are some obvious hormonal issues, but there are many other ways your hormone system reveals it is out of balance, such as thyroid, adrenal, and testosterone issues. Whatever your specific hormonal imbalance, the tools in this toolbox can help get your system back in order by reducing inflammation to improve hormone receptor activity and brain-hormonal communication (in the hypothalamic-pituitary-adrenal, thyroid, or gonadal axes). Even when you are in a period of hormonal upheaval such as perimenopause, you should notice major symptom improvement on this plan. This toolbox will help get you back on track fast.

1. Sole water. This electrolyte-infused water supports the adrenal hormone aldosterone,[37] which is partially responsible for electrolyte and fluid balance. It stabilizes sodium levels and is easy to make. Once you have made it, it won't take more than a few seconds to add it to your daily routine. To make it, find a large mason jar (any large size— you can find these online if you don't have any) with a plastic lid—a metal lid can oxidize and corrode when it comes into contact with salt water—and fill it a quarter of the way up with high-quality sea salt, Celtic salt, or Himalayan pink salt, or a mixture or combination of these three. Add filtered water but leave a little room at the top. Put on the lid, shake it up, and let it sit overnight. In the morning, check your sole water. If you can see some salt in the bottom of the jar, the water is saturated with the salt. If you don't see any salt, add a teaspoon more. Shake, and give it an hour to dissolve. Keep going until some salt remains at the bottom. When the sole water is fully saturated, it is ready. Add 1 teaspoon to a glass of water every morning and drink it before eating anything. Dip only plastic or wood into the water to scoop it out—no metal utensils.

2. Sea vegetables. Plant foods from the sea—for example, kelp, nori, dulse, kombu, wakame, and agar—are high in iodine, which you need to produce thyroid hormones. Every cell needs thyroid hormones to function properly.

3. Wild-caught fish—specifically salmon, mackerel, and sardines. These are rich in vitamin D, which supports hundreds of different metabolic pathways, and contain healthy fats that support hormone balance.[38]

4. Chasteberry supplements. This berry naturally supports healthy progesterone levels to balance out your ratio of progesterone to estrogen.[39]

5. Rooibos tea. This bright red tea from the African red bush supports adrenal function by balancing cortisol, one of the stress hormones.

6. Ashwagandha supplements. The ultimate cortisol balancer, this herb, popular in Ayurvedic medicine therapy, supports the hypothalamic-pituitary-adrenal (HPA) axis and the thyroid by boosting sluggish thyroid hormones, and helps you feel calm, especially when you have been suffering from mood swings and/or hormone-fueled anxiety.[40] [41]

7. Evening primrose oil supplements. This oil contains the hormone-supporting omega-6 fatty acids GLA and LA, and helps relieve symptoms of menopause, PMS, PCOS, and hormonally fueled acne.[42]

8. Schisandra powder. This berry supports the adrenals and is good to add to smoothies or teas.

Mantra: *My hormones are in perfect harmony. I am in perfect harmony.*

Repeat this mantra aloud or in your mind as it occurs to you, and for 5 to 15 minutes while sitting quietly in the morning and/or evening. It will help with both physical and mental balance.

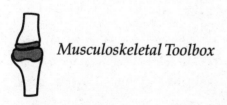 *Musculoskeletal Toolbox*

Inflammation in the structures that hold your body together can have a wide range of painful effects—from tight, sore muscles and joints to osteoarthritis, fibromyalgia, and autoimmune diseases that settle in the joints (such as rheumatoid arthritis, Sjögren's syndrome, and lupus). It can also compromise joint, muscle, and connective tissue structure, making you too loose and more prone to injury or too tight with more pain and stiffness. If you don't decrease inflammation in these areas, you could end up with a chronic pain problem, an inability to exercise, or even a disability due to joint damage and muscle weakness. This toolbox targets the areas that give your body structure and provides it with the ability to move and function better, to get you moving comfortably again. Here are your tools.

1. MSM (methylsulfonylmethane) supplements. This sulfur-containing compound reduces joint and muscle pain through its natural anti-inflammatory action.[43]

2. Turmeric. This ancient medicinal spice is one of the most potent anti-inflammatory spices, due to the curcuminoids and other beneficial compounds it contains.

3. Collagen powder. This powder, which you can add to smoothies or any hot or cold drink, is restorative for connective tissue.

4. Glucosamine sulfate (with or without chondroitin sulfate). This supplement supports healthy cartilage and synovial fluid to restore joint health, reduce pain, and calm inflammation. Studies show it has legitimate pain-reducing and mobility-increasing effects.[44]

5. Infrared sauna. This type of sauna in particular reduces inflammation and can feel relaxing and stress-reducing (unless you are intolerant to heat).[45]

6. Cryotherapy. This therapy uses deep cold temperatures for short time periods to drive down inflammation levels.[46] It is rejuvenating and can result in significant pain relief (unless you are intolerant to cold).

7. Massage. Do you need another excuse to make massage a part of your regular routine? Various techniques, especially Swedish, trigger point, myofascial release, and deep-tissue techniques, target and relieve muscle pain and tension.[47] [48]

8. CBD oil. This oil from the hemp or cannabis plant helps alleviate pain in the musculoskeletal system. Don't worry (or maybe I should say, "Sorry, but . . ."), CBD is refined so it does not contain any (or contains very little) THC. You won't get high, but you will get pain relief.[49]

> **Mantra:** *I have the power to release my pain and capture the health that I deserve.*

Repeat this mantra aloud or in your mind whenever you think of it throughout the day, and for 5 to 15 minutes while sitting quietly in the morning and/or evening. Mantra meditation relaxes muscle tension and relieves pain.

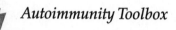 *Autoimmunity Toolbox*

In America alone, it's estimated that 50 million people have been diagnosed with an autoimmune disease. In most cases, the official diagnostic criterion is that the patient's immune system has already destroyed a significant amount of their body—for instance, there has to be 90 percent destruction of the adrenal glands for autoimmune adrenal issues or Addison's disease to be diagnosed. There also has to be major destruction of the neurological and digestive systems in a diagnosis of neurological autoimmunity like multiple sclerosis (MS), or gut autoimmunity, like celiac disease.

This amount of autoimmune-inflammation attack does not happen overnight—it's the end stage of the larger autoimmune-inflammation spectrum. My focus is on addressing the causes of the inflammation before the patient reaches that end-stage level of destruction.

There are three main stages of the autoimmune-inflammation spectrum:

1. Silent Autoimmunity: There are positive antibody labs but no noticeable symptoms.

2. Autoimmune Reactivity: There are positive antibody labs and the patient is experiencing symptoms.

3. Autoimmune Disease: There's enough body destruction to be diagnosed and loads of potential symptoms.

In my functional medicine center, I see many people in the second stage: not sick enough to have been slapped with a diagnosis code, but nonetheless feeling the effects of autoimmune reactivity. People living somewhere on the inflammation spectrum often get sent from to doctor to doctor, with a pile of labs and medications, yet nothing to show for it. These patients are often essentially told, "Well, you will probably get lupus in a few years—come back then."

Inflammation is a major factor for most, if not all, autoimmune diseases. Autoimmunity is a condition in which the immune system attacks its own tissues, thinking they are foreign invaders (like viruses or bacteria are). What once used to be a rare condition is now common, with approximately a hundred different recognized autoimmune diseases and another forty conditions that have an autoimmune component. I suspect these numbers will continue to rise as we discover more about how various diseases operate. Some of the more common ones I see are rheumatoid arthritis, systemic lupus erythematosus, inflammatory bowel disorders, celiac disease, psoriasis, scleroderma, vitiligo, pernicious anemia, Hashimoto's thyroiditis, Addison's disease, Graves' disease, Sjögren's syndrome, type 1 diabetes, hidradenitis suppurativa, and multiple sclerosis (MS).

Most often, the immune system attacks the digestive system, joints, muscles, skin, connective tissue, brain and spinal cord, endocrine glands (such as the thyroid and adrenals), and/or blood vessels. These diseases can be mild in some and debilitating, even fatal, in others. If you already have an autoimmune disease, this toolbox will help support your health. If you are not diagnosed but the quiz suggested your immune-centered inflammation is advancing, cooling inflammation is crucial, and you have no time to lose! Start with this toolbox.

1. **Organ meats** from grass-fed or pastured animals. Once a common part of the human diet, organ meats are much less common now, especially in the United States, but they contain some of the highest amounts of true vitamin A, bioavailable B vitamins, and minerals like iron of any food. Vitamin A deficiencies are linked to autoimmune conditions, and organ meats can replenish deficiencies quickly.

2. **Extra-virgin cod-liver oil.** This ultra-healthy fat is rich in fat-soluble vitamins, which the immune system requires to stay healthy and function appropriately.

3. **Emu oil.** This oil from the ostrich-like emu is rich in vitamin K_2, which helps balance the important family of enzymes called iNOS (inducible nitric oxide synthases) to modulate inflammatory pathways.

4. **Broccoli sprouts.** These sprouts have some of the highest levels of methylation-supporting sulforaphane, which can dramatically reduce inflammation and maintain proper T-cell function.[50]

5. **Elderberry.** This fruit helps balance the immune system.[51] Elderberry is typically found in a liquid supplement form.

6. **Black cumin seed oil.** This supplement increases T-regulatory cells to rebalance an out-of-control immune system and lower inflammation.[52]

7. **Pterostilbene supplements.** This compound, which is similar to resveratrol, decreases inflammatory NF-κB proteins and increases the anti-inflammatory Nrf2 pathway.[53]

8. Water or coconut kefir. These fermented drinks contain naturally occurring vitamin K_2 as a by-product of the fermentation process. They also contain kefiran, a unique sugar produced by kefir grains that has the ability to decrease inflammation and calm the immune system.[54]

Mantra: *My body is powerful and constantly restores itself.*

Repeat this mantra aloud or in your mind whenever you think of it throughout the day, and for 5 to 15 minutes while sitting quietly in the morning and/or evening. Reducing stress also reduces inflammation.

Polyinflammation Toolbox

Multiple areas of inflammation are a sign that your health is significantly compromised. Are you facing a future of imminent chronic disease if you don't change course? Maybe. Or maybe you already have a diagnosis. In any case, this is no time to dabble in the next fun fad diet. You must do something dramatically different to see different results. If you have been waiting for the right time to make a drastic change for your health, it's now. Let's get serious because your health may be at stake, and the power to change that is in your hands. Fortunately, you have quite a few toolboxes at your disposal—in fact, all of them! Dip into all the toolboxes that are relevant to your particular areas of inflammation. You could focus on the toolboxes for the areas you are most concerned about, or you could try strategies from a different toolbox every day. If you are having a bad joint day, go to the musculoskeletal toolbox and pick some medicinal foods and therapies. If your digestion seems off, check out the digestive toolbox to try some digestive food medicines and therapies. If it's a nasty brain fog day, head on over to the brain/nervous system toolbox and sample some of those therapies. Browse freely, use all the tools you can, and tackle that inflammation like you mean business!

Mantra: *I reclaim my vitality.*

Repeat this mantra aloud or in your mind whenever you think of it throughout the day, and for 5 to 15 minutes while sitting quietly in the morning and/or evening. This one sentiment is at the heart of everything you are doing on the Elimin8 plan.

Time-Restricted Feeding: A Tool for All

Intermittent fasting (IF) or time-restricted feeding (TRF) is something anyone can try. Throughout human history, food was not as constantly and excessively available as it is now. People couldn't always eat whenever they felt like it. Our bodies adapted to this and they respond favorably—not to starvation, but to periods of not eating or of eating less. Both IF and TRF protocols[55] are a great way to lower inflammation and enhance something called autophagy. Autophagy is your body's ability to clean out dead, dysfunctional cells and lower inflammation levels. Three simple ways you can enhance your diet, whether you are practicing an elimination diet or not, are eating between eight A.M. and six P.M. only or between twelve noon to six P.M. only, or skipping a meal each day or periodically. For more advanced intermittent fasting protocols, check out my book *Ketotarian*.

Remember to keep your toolbox close to remind you of the foods and therapies that can benefit your goal of reducing your inflammation, no matter where you are on the inflammation spectrum. Now it's time to begin the actual plan by stepping down over the course of four or eight days (depending on your track), giving up a few things at a time until you are 100 percent compliant. I'll help you, step by step, to eliminate confusion. Let's jump right in!

4

INITI8: TRANSITIONING INTO THE ELIMINATION PHASE

Now that you have chosen your Core4 or Elimin8 track and you have your bio-individualized toolbox, it's time to begin the actual process of eliminating inflammatory foods from your life. We'll start by phasing out the four (for the Core4 track) or eight (for the Elimin8 track) eliminated items I gave you in the previous chapter, one at a time.

Although you may be tempted to ditch everything at once just to get going faster, I find that for many people, drastic changes all at once are often overwhelming. Enthusiasm can turn to frustration when the change is too sudden, so I prefer this step-down approach. Wellness shouldn't be stressful. There is magic in leaning in to new things. Give yourself grace and lightness during this time and always. Focus on all the delicious, inflammation-calming foods in the next chapter that you get to enjoy. This Initi8 phase allows you to ease into the program in a more thoughtful, sustainable way. Even on the first day, as you eliminate the very first food, you can become more self-aware. Start by observing how the removal of each food affects you initially. This is an important part of body awareness and sensitivity to your individual reactions.

THE STEP-DOWN PROCESS

Over the course of the next four or eight days, you will step down into full elimination mode. Whether you are doing the Core4 or Elimin8 track, your first four days will be the same. You will be giving up one Core4 food each day. After four days, Core4 people can move on to the next chapter. Elimin8 people will keep going for four more days, eliminating four more inflammatory foods. After eight days, the Elimin8 people will be ready to move on to the next chapter.

Information about what to do as you give up each inflammatory food—including why to give it up, how to give it up, and what to eat instead—comes after the charts.

Core4 Track Step-Down Schedule

DAY	FOOD TO ELIMINATE
1	All grains: Wheat, barley, rye, rice, quinoa, corn, etc.
2	Dairy products: Milk, yogurt, cheese, cream, etc., from cows, goats, or sheep
3	All added sweeteners: White and brown sugar, high-fructose corn syrup, maple syrup, honey, coconut sugar, agave nectar, stevia, monk fruit, sugar alcohols, etc.
4	Inflammatory oils: Corn, soybean, canola, sunflower, grapeseed, vegetable, etc.

Elimin8 Track Step-Down Schedule

DAY	FOOD TO ELIMINATE
1	All grains: Wheat, barley, rye, rice, quinoa, corn, etc.
2	Dairy products: Milk, yogurt, cheese, cream, etc., from cows, goats, or sheep
3	All added sweeteners: White and brown sugar, high-fructose corn syrup, maple syrup, honey, coconut sugar, agave nectar, etc.

4	Inflammatory oils: Corn, soybean, canola, sunflower, grapeseed, vegetable oil, etc.
5	Legumes: Lentils, black beans, pinto beans, white beans, soybeans, tofu, lima beans, chickpeas, peanuts, peanut butter, etc.
6	Nuts and seeds: Almonds, walnuts, pecans, sunflower seeds, pumpkin seeds, sesame seeds, chia seeds, nut and seed butters, etc.
7	Eggs, whites and yolks
8	Nightshades: Tomatoes, white and yellow potatoes, eggplant, all peppers, etc.

Day One for Core4 and Elimin8: Grains

Although grains are beloved by many, even to the point of addiction for some of us, grains are one of the foods most likely to be causing you inflammation and compromising your digestive integrity. That is why it is so important that we get them out . . . for now. You will have the opportunity to reintroduce grains later if you really want to bring them back into your diet, but let's cool your inflammation first so we can get a true reading on how your body genuinely responds to grain.

We live in a grain-centric society. Grains are the foundation of meals for many people. If you have ever looked at the contents of other people's shopping carts at the supermarket, you may have noticed that they are mostly filled with grains, grains, and more grains: cereal for breakfast, a sandwich for lunch, and a grain as a side (at least), if not the main course (hello, spaghetti), for dinner. Grains are the backbone of industrial farming and are a multibillion-dollar juggernaut. Grain lobbies have a lot of political power. Grains are even the foundation of the famous food pyramid of old (or a huge slice of the USDA MyPlate). It's no surprise, then, that even the idea of eliminating grains sounds radical to many. However, a grain-free diet is hardly radical. Heavy grain consumption is a relatively recent dietary adoption for humans.[1] Let's look at the many good reasons to ditch grains for more nutrient-dense alternatives.

....

The Celiac Spectrum

Researchers are now finding evidence for what we've been saying for decades in functional medicine: Mild food reactivities like gluten sensitivity with only occasional, mostly tolerable symptoms are on one end of the larger inflammation spectrum, with autoimmune diseases like celiac disease (CD) on the opposite side.[2] I believe that just as there is an autoimmune-inflammation spectrum, there is a spectrum from mild gluten sensitivity to true celiac disease.[3] I call this the celiac spectrum.

Conventional doctors can diagnose you with celiac disease or tell you that you don't have celiac disease, based on the level of destruction of the microvilli in your small intestine. Recently, however, doctors are beginning to admit that some of those without diagnosable celiac disease do seem to suffer with legitimate, significant symptoms when they eat gluten. Also, I'm not completely convinced that the diagnostic criteria for celiac disease are sufficiently inclusive. For example, only about 10 percent of people with celiac disease have obvious GI symptoms.[4] Instead, they experience other seemingly unrelated symptoms like anxiety, depression, or skin problems. Estimates are that only about 5 percent of celiacs are ever diagnosed,[5] largely because doctors usually suspect celiac disease only in patients with digestive issues (and even then, they often don't test for it). This means that around 3 million Americans with celiac disease have no idea that they have it.

If you discover through the process in this book (or if you already know) that you get symptoms after eating gluten, then you are on the gluten sensitivity/celiac spectrum, and you should avoid all gluten for the rest of your life. For now, I also recommend giving up all grains, because the inflammatory effect from even non-gluten grains can aggravate symptoms in many people. If you have a diagnosed food sensitivity or autoimmune condition like celiac disease, reducing all grains can be helpful in bringing down overall inflammation. If this is you, I also suggest jumping right into the Elimin8 track for maximum effect.

....

WHY GIVE THEM UP (FOR NOW): Here are some good reasons why grains have got to go:

- **Gluten.** It's nearly impossible not to hear the G-word thrown around these days. An explosion of gluten research has shed light on this protein in wheat, rye, barley, and spelt—conservative estimates approximate that 1 in 20 Americans have gluten intolerance. Gluten is difficult to digest compared to the proteins in other grains, so its presence in the digestive tract can inflame the intestinal lining, loosening the tight junctions and contributing to leaky gut syndrome. When this happens, undigested food proteins such as gluten and bacterial endotoxins called lipopolysaccharides (LPS) can pass into the bloodstream, creating an inflammatory reaction outside the GI tract that could trigger an autoimmune response.

- **Lectins.** Lectins are proteins found most abundantly in grains, legumes, nuts, seeds, nightshades (tomatoes, peppers, eggplant, and potatoes), and squash (mainly the skin and seeds). These plant defense mechanisms are indigestible, and like gluten, lectins can cause digestive problems and trigger inflammation in many people,[6] compromising the intestinal barrier. Lectins can also bind to insulin[7] and leptin[8] receptor sites, fueling hormonal resistance patterns.

- **Enzyme inhibitors.** Your body makes enzymes to assist with digestion, but grains contain alpha-amylase inhibitors and protease inhibitors, which can inhibit these digestive enzymes, causing digestive difficulties for you if you are sensitive.

- **Phytic acid and phytates.** These compounds are anti-nutrients[9] that bind to minerals like calcium and iron in your body, making them unusable to you. Mineral deficiencies like osteoporosis can be perpetuated by the presence of phytates.

- **Saponins.** Pseudo-grains like quinoa are particularly high in these anti-nutrients,[10] which can contribute to inflammation and gut permeability in sensitive people.

- **Sugars.** Grains are high in sugars, which can cause blood sugar and insulin spikes and could lead to insulin resistance, metabolic syndrome, prediabetes, and type 2 diabetes in susceptible people.

- **High omega-6 levels.** Fats are essential for optimal health, but there are inflammatory fats and anti-inflammatory fats. Grains are high in polyunsaturated omega-6 fats, which are inflammatory when out of proportion to omega-3 fats. Since most people eat far more omega-6 fats, grains can contribute to this imbalance.

It is also important to remember that grains have changed from their original forms due to crossbreeding, hybridization, genetic modification, and the frequent use of agricultural chemicals (like glyphosate) on grain crops. You don't need grains to get fiber, and vegetables and fruits are far more nutrient dense than grains, without the harmful effects of gluten, lectins, enzyme inhibitors, phytic acid, omega-6 fatty acids, and all the other negative aspects I've already mentioned. You need not fear that you will become "grain deficient." There is no such thing.

In the Reintegr8 stage, when your inflammation has cooled, you may notice that you are able to tolerate some grains and not others. If you want to bring back grains, giving them up for a while is the only way to get an accurate reading on your body's response.

HOW TO GIVE THEM UP: Stop eating all foods made with wheat, barley, rye, spelt, oats, rice, corn, quinoa, and any other grain. That means no bread, pasta, cereal, or baked goods like muffins and cookies. This may seem impossible at first, especially if your diet is currently grain-heavy, but don't worry—there are still lots of delicious anti-inflammatory foods for you to eat!

GRAINS TO ELIMINATE

- Wheat, including wheat berries, bulgur wheat (as in tabbouleh salad), and Cream of Wheat, as well as anything made with wheat (like wheat beer) or wheat flour, including white flour and whole wheat flour: most types of bread, pasta (durum and semolina are types of wheat), bagels, English muffins, cake, cookies, doughnuts, etc.

■ Barley (often in soup) and anything made with barley, including most beer.

■ Rye, including anything made with rye, such as rye bread and rye whiskey.

■ Spelt and anything made with spelt, such as spelt pretzels and spelt bread.

■ Oats, including oatmeal and anything made with oat flour, like oat bread, granola, and muesli.

■ Rice, including brown, white, red, basmati, jasmine, and sushi rice.

■ Corn, including fresh corn and anything made with corn, such as cornmeal, corn tortillas, and corn chips.

■ All other grains, including the so-called ancient grains: quinoa, millet, amaranth, Kamut, einkorn, etc.

GRAIN-FREE FOODS TO INCORPORATE

■ Instead of toast in the morning, try eating an avocado sprinkled with salt and pepper. Scoop it out with a spoon.

■ Green smoothies are quick, nutrient-dense options for people in a hurry, or for those who don't like to eat a lot for breakfast. If you are doing the Core4 track only, another good breakfast option is eggs.

■ For sandwiches, use lettuce wraps, collard leaves, or mushroom caps in place of bread, buns, and tortillas.

- Sweet potatoes can be made into chips or fries for that starchy taste you may be craving or mash them for a starchy side dish.

- Vegetable chips can be made from thick leafy greens like kale or sliced root vegetables like carrots, beets, and cassava. I also like cassava tortillas.

- Plantains make great chips. Try them for delicious South American–style "nachos."

- Try baking with grain-free flours like coconut flour, almond flour, arrowroot powder, tapioca starch, plantain flour, cassava flour, and tigernut flour. (There are many good grain-free baking books available.)

Day Two for Core4 and Elimin8: Dairy Products

Maybe you grew up thinking milk was the best for you. It has protein and calcium, and because so many of us associate milk with childhood nutrition, it *seems* like it must be a healthy food. However, for many people and for many reasons, dairy is inflammatory. While high-quality organic milk from grass-fed cows not treated with growth hormones and antibiotics may be great for your system, I find that many of my patients feel better without dairy in their diets. Some do report that while cow's milk gives them reactions, they do fine on goat milk, sheep milk, or camel milk (yeah, it's a thing). While these milks also contain lactose (the sugar that naturally occurs in milk, which gives many people gastrointestinal issues), milks from animals other than cows do have a different type of casein (a milk protein) that is easier to digest. For now, however, you will step away from all animal-based dairy products to give your system a rest. You will determine, after the elimination period, whether certain dairy products work for you or not.

How do you live without your fancy French goat cheese, your post-workout whey protein shake, or your morning Greek yogurt?

Not to worry. There are plenty of delicious and widely available "dairy" products made from plants that can see you through.

WHY GIVE IT UP (FOR NOW): There are all kinds of reasons people might react to dairy products like milk, ice cream, yogurt, cream, and cheese.

- **Lactose.** Those who are intolerant of lactose (milk sugar) lack the enzyme to digest dairy products containing lactose. In these people, eating dairy products can cause uncomfortable digestive problems, from bloating and gas to diarrhea.

- **Casein and/or whey.** Those who can digest lactose without a problem may have a different issue—they may be intolerant of or sensitive to the proteins in milk—specifically, casein and whey. The casein molecule can look a lot like the gluten molecule to an overreactive immune system, so bodies that are sensitive to one are often sensitive to the other, causing inflammation in the digestive tract. If casein proteins pass through the protective gut lining due to intestinal permeability, they could trigger more serious reactions, like autoimmunity. In people with casein or whey intolerance or sensitivity, dairy products can also cause severe digestive problems, like stomach cramps and diarrhea, as well as other seemingly unrelated effects, like breathing problems, vomiting, hives, joint pain, extreme fatigue, neurological symptoms, and behavioral changes (or even anaphylaxis in people who are allergic to the casein or whey protein in milk).

- **Additives.** Want growth hormone with your milk? Conventional milk available in supermarkets often comes from cows injected with bovine growth hormone, which dairy farmers administer to increase milk production. We don't yet know what effect this could have on the people who drink it, immediately or in the long run, but I do not advise ingesting these hormones, which I consider to be xenobiotics—substances foreign to the human body. Also, dairy cows are often pumped full of antibiotics to prevent or treat mastitis, which develops as a result of irritation or infection from the milking machines. That means you could get an extra dose of residual antibiotics, and probably a little mastitis pus, in every glass of cow's milk. Yummy.

- **Added sugar.** Of course flavored milks like chocolate milk are loaded with added sweeteners, which you will be giving up tomorrow anyway.

··

Know Your Cows: A1 and A2 Casein

There are two main kinds of casein protein. The A1 subtype[11] of casein is most common in the United States. It is the type of casein produced by cows from northern Europe, such as Holstein and Friesian breeds. Although the research is not yet definitive, emerging studies suggest that milk with more A1 casein[12] tends to be more inflammatory and difficult to digest, and it may even contribute to certain health issues like diabetes and heart disease.

Then there's the more ancient A2 casein. A2 is the subtype in the milk of cows that originally come from southern France and the Channel Islands, such as Guernsey and Jersey cows—many of which are now producing milk in New Zealand and France. According to preliminary research (and personal reports from many of my patients), milk with more A2 casein is less inflammatory and easier to digest. It may also be richer in nutrients. While most conventional dairy products are not currently labeled with their casein type, as more people learn about this differentiation, more companies are labeling A2 in their products. If you do decide to try to reintroduce dairy products after the elimination phase of this book, look for dairy products made from milk that comes from A2 cow breeds, or milk produced in New Zealand and France as well as Africa and India. For now, we are eliminating both A2 and A1 dairy, but keep in mind that many people tolerate grass-fed A2 dairy (especially fermented products like cheese and yogurt) when they reintroduce it.

··

HOW TO GIVE IT UP: Get all milk, ice cream, yogurt, cheese (ouch, I know . . .), and anything else containing lactose or casein out of your diet, whether it comes from a cow, a goat, a sheep, a cat, or any other animal.

DAIRY FOODS TO ELIMINATE

Eliminate any of the following if they come from cows, goats, sheep, horses, camels . . . all the beasts.

- Milk
- Butter (but ghee, which is clarified butter with the dairy proteins removed, is fine)
- Cream
- Yogurt
- Ice cream
- Cheese

WHAT TO EAT INSTEAD: Fortunately, there are tons of anti-inflammatory plant milk products available, made of gluten-free grains like nuts, seeds, or coconuts. (For those on the Elimin8 track, nut and seed milks are okay for now, but you will eliminate these in a few days. Use them as dairy transition products, if necessary. Coconut milk products will continue to be okay for you.) Nondairy yogurt, cheese, and ice cream have all improved a lot in the last few years, so if you haven't tried these in a while, give them another try. You may find you don't even miss the cow juice.

DAIRY-FREE FOODS TO INCORPORATE

Look for plant-based versions of milk. If you are doing the Core4 track, check out milk made from coconuts, almonds, cashews, hazelnuts, hempseed or any other nut or seed, or peas. Cheese made from nuts—new artisanal brands, especially of spreadable cream-cheese-like products—can be virtually indistinguishable from dairy cheese. If you are doing the Elimin8 track, you can have nut milk for now, but products made with coconut are always a good dairy alternative for you. Coconuts contain just the kind of fat your brain will love.

Day Three for Core4 and Elimin8: All Added Sweeteners

This one is a no-brainer—because too much sugar *literally* inflames your brain, causing impaired cognitive function and worse memory.[13] I'm pretty sure you like your brain and want it to keep working into old age. So let's get the sugar out.

WHY GIVE THEM UP (FOR NOW): There are mountains of studies proving that refined sugars, such as white sugar, brown sugar, high-fructose corn syrup (or any corn syrup), and similar cheap sweeteners cause inflammation in almost everybody and can increase your risk of many chronic diseases, including diabetes, liver disease, and heart disease,[14] (sugar increases your chance of dying from heart disease, even if you aren't overweight[15]). Artificial sweeteners can be even worse, toying with your gut bacteria and tipping your scales to make you weigh more,[16] even though you may have thought your calorie-free beverage choice was doing the opposite. Even natural sweeteners keep you focused on that sweet taste, instead of refining your palate to appreciate the natural sweetness of foods.

Sugar is addictive. The average American consumes about 3,550 pounds of sugar in a lifetime—the equivalent of 1.7 million Skittles, or an industrial-sized dumpster full of white sugar. We are going to ignore that dumpster and keep all added sweeteners out of your body for now. Later, you may find you can reintegrate some natural sweeteners, but you won't know for sure if you tolerate them unless you give them up for a while.

HOW TO GIVE THEM UP: Quitting sugar is a little bit like quitting smoking. Sometimes you have to go cold turkey. You might have intense cravings at first, but hold on and don't give in to them. Within a few days, the craving should subside, or at least get much easier to resist.

ADDED SWEETENERS TO ELIMINATE

- **White or brown sugar,** in all forms and for all purposes, from your morning tea to baked goods like cookies and cake.

- **Any syrup,** such as corn syrup, high-fructose corn syrup, maple syrup, brown rice syrup, agave nectar, honey, and date syrup.

- **Any natural sweetener,** including coconut sugar, date sugar, maple sugar, corn sugar, evaporated cane juice, cane juice crystals, beet sugar, stevia, monk fruit, sugar alcohols like xylitol, and concentrated fruit juice.

- Anything containing **artificial sweeteners,** including aspartame (brand names like Equal and NutraSweet), saccharin (in Sweet'N Low), sucralose (in Splenda), and acesulfame K (in Sunett and Sweet One).

- **Any packaged food with added sweeteners** in the ingredients list. Sugar goes by many names—not just the sugars and syrups listed above, but caramel, corn sweetener, corn syrup solids, fructose, dextrose, dextrin, glucose, maltose, maltodextrin, sucrose . . . anything ending in -ose.

- **Candy.** All candy.

- **Soda, diet soda, energy drinks, and bottled fruit drinks.**

- **Most desserts**—cake, cookies, cheesecake, brownies, pie, pudding, etc., purchased or homemade. Sugar is also often added to dried fruit, and sugar and/or artificial sweetener is almost always present in flavored yogurt, granola bars, and breakfast cereal. You can have unsweetened dried fruit and unsweetened nondairy yogurt (such as plain coconut yogurt).

■ **Hidden sweetener in nonsweet foods**, like ketchup, barbecue sauce, pasta sauce, soup, crackers, salad dressing, canned fruit, deli salads (like coleslaw and broccoli salad), bottled tea, and much more. Read the label and get sugar-savvy.

WHAT TO EAT INSTEAD: There are so many delicious sweet options in nature, like fresh fruit (nature's candy), root vegetables (especially sweet potatoes and yams), coconut, and even some natural spices, like cinnamon and anise, as well as sweet-tasting but unsweetened herbal teas. Unsweetened dried fruit is fine, too, but don't overdo it, as the natural fruit sugars are concentrated by the drying process. For some people, it's better to stay away from all sweet foods for a while, to break the palate of its bad habit.

In a few days, as your taste buds recover from the overstimulation of refined sugar and become more sensitive (this happens more quickly in some and takes longer in others), natural foods will taste much sweeter. Some are fine with natural sweeteners and are able to eat these in moderation. If this is you—or if you absolutely *need* sweetness today and you can't go a minute longer—try anything on the following list. If you don't have a craving for sweets, then see if you can go without eating anything sweet and see how you feel.

NATURALLY SWEETENED FOODS TO INCORPORATE

Sweet fresh and dried fruits are a treat, but it's good to enjoy them in moderation. Have all the sweet herbs, herbal teas (no sweetener added, of course), and other naturally sweet whole foods you like, such as:

- **Raw or dried (unsweetened) coconut.**

- **Raw cacao nibs or carob.** Sprinkle them on a halved banana with a little coconut—like a candy bar, but so much better. Look out for any added sugar.

- **Sweet herbs and spices**—cinnamon, anise, allspice, cardamom, cloves, coriander, fennel, mint, basil, or tarragon.

- **Herbal teas.** Many are naturally sweet.

- **Still or sparkling water flavored with fresh fruit.**

Day Four for Core4 and Elimin8: Inflammatory Oils

You may have been told that vegetable oils are better for you than animal fats, but this is not the case.[17] The truth is that processed industrial seed and grain oils like corn oil, canola oil, and that mysterious "vegetable oil" are inflammatory.

WHY GIVE THEM UP (FOR NOW): To extract these oils, the seeds are subjected to high temperatures. Then the oils are removed with petroleum solvents and further chemically treated to remove the by-products of the process. Next they are often colored and scented so they don't smell like what they really are—the unnatural result of an aggressive chemical process. These oils also frequently contain artificial antioxidants like BHA and BHT to keep them shelf-stable for long periods of time. Mmm, old oil . . .

Vegetable oils also contain more polyunsaturated fatty acids than oils from olives and coconuts (more naturally extracted through good old-fashioned pressing). These polyunsaturated fats oxidize easily, so these oils are often major sources of inflammatory free radicals, especially when heated. We'll be sticking with more natural, anti-inflammatory oils like cold-pressed olive oil, avocado oil, coconut oil, and ghee (clarified butter with the dairy solids removed) for the rest of the Elimin8 program.

HOW TO GIVE THEM UP: There is no need to give up all oil

or added fat. There are good oils and there are bad oils. All you have to do is know the difference and stick to the good ones. If you've been using a lot of industrial seed oil, your inflammation level will respond quickly with this switch.

INFLAMMATORY OILS TO ELIMINATE

- Corn oil
- Canola oil
- Sunflower oil
- Soybean oil
- Cottonseed oil
- Safflower oil
- Grapeseed oil
- Rice bran oil
- Vegetable oil
- Margarines and "buttery spreads"
- Most packaged foods containing any fat. Read the label.

WHAT TO EAT INSTEAD: There are bad oils and there are good oils, and the difference couldn't be more dramatic. The bad oils are inflammatory, but the good oils are anti-inflammatory and infuse your body with nutrients and brain-boosting fats that balance hormones and are good for every system. Some are best served in their raw state, like extra-virgin olive oil, and others are good for cooking, like coconut oil or avocado oil.

ANTI-INFLAMMATORY OILS TO INCORPORATE

Cold-pressed oils, to enjoy raw (don't use these for cooking):

- Extra-virgin olive oil
- Extra-virgin avocado oil
- Extra-virgin coconut oil

Oils and fats for cooking:

- Avocado oil

- Olive oil (not extra virgin)

- Coconut oil

- Grass-fed ghee (clarified butter—this comes from milk, but because the lactose and casein are no longer present, it is fine to eat on both the Elimin8 and Core4 tracks)

- Palm shortening (organic only)

Core4 Track people, stop here. You can move on to the next chapter. Elimin8 folks, stay with me! You've got just four more days to go.

Day Five for Elimin8: Legumes

Legumes—the bean and pea family, including peanuts and soybeans—have a variety of qualities that can make them inflammatory for some people. They contain lectins and phytic acid, which can trigger inflammation and interfere with mineral absorption.[18] In the case of peanuts, there is also the possibility of aflatoxin mold contamination. Lectins are part of the defense mechanism of plants.[19] On average, 15 percent of a legume's proteins are lectins. Our immune systems have evolved to create antibodies that protect us from lectins, but not all of us have the genetics that effectively create enough antibodies to protect us from every kind of lectin.[20] This is why some of us are more sensitive to the lectins in foods than others. You will be able to test your tolerance to legumes during reintroduction.

NOTE: If you are a vegan or a vegetarian, strongly consider bringing animal products such as wild-caught fish back into your diet, at least for the duration of the Elimin8 program (but this isn't required—see my discussion of doing this elimination diet as a vegetarian or vegan on page 61).

LEGUMES TO ELIMINATE

- All beans, including pinto, black, white, red, navy, kidney, lima, fava, garbanzo, and mung beans

- All lentils

- Soy and all products made with soy, including edamame, tofu, miso, soy sauce, and soy-based tempeh

- Any packaged or processed foods and protein powders containing any ingredients that contain the word soy, such as soy protein isolate.

- Peanuts and all peanut products, including peanut butter and peanut sauce

NOTE: Fresh peas and beans that come in pods, like green beans, green peas, and snow peas, are okay to eat.

LEGUME-FREE FOODS TO INCORPORATE

- Starchy vegetables can have a similar texture to cooked beans. Add cubed sweet potatoes, turnips, or rutabaga to soup or chili, or try them mashed in place of refried beans—good with tacos.

- Mushrooms—all types; whole, sliced, or chopped—make a meaty, hearty addition to foods and a great legume replacement.

Day Six for Elimin8: Nuts and Seeds

Nuts and seeds can be difficult to digest for some people. They contain lectins and roughage that can irritate the digestive tract and immune systems of some people.[21] Another potential issue with nuts and seeds is the conventional roasting and industrial seed oils that are added to store-bought varieties. Consuming oxidized oils can cause even more inflammation. Note: If you were including almond or other nut milk in your diet up to this point as you transitioned away from dairy products, today is the day to move to coconut-milk-based dairy alternatives only, if you still feel that you need a milk substitute.

NUTS AND SEEDS TO ELIMINATE

Nuts

- Acorns (for any squirrel that is reading this)
- Almonds
- Brazil nuts
- Cashews
- Chestnuts
- Hazelnuts
- Hickory nuts
- Kola nuts
- Macadamia nuts
- Pecans
- Pili nuts
- Pine nuts
- Pistachios
- Sacha inchi
- Walnuts

Seeds

- Chia
- Flax
- Hemp
- Poppy
- Pumpkin
- Sesame
- Safflower
- Sunflower

NUT- AND SEED-FREE FOODS TO INCORPORATE

In any recipe that includes nuts or seeds, or for easy snacking, try the following as a replacement:

- Dried coconut flakes or shreds (unsweetened)

- Dried blueberries, tart cherries, or currants (unsweetened)

- Cassava chips

- Plantain chips

- Tigernuts (these are actually small root vegetables, not nuts)

- Dried banana chips

- Roasted vegetable "chips," dried in a dehydrator or low-temperature oven (try kale, thinly sliced squash, or thinly sliced root vegetables)

- Nutritional yeast, in savory recipes, for a cheesy flavor

Day Seven for Elimin8: Eggs

Many people, me included, eat eggs without any problem. For some people, however, the albumin in egg whites can be inflammatory, particularly for those with autoimmune conditions. In fact, that egg white omelet you thought was so healthy may be something your body cannot tolerate. Egg whites are a common source of food sensitivity, but for some, the whole egg is a problem, too. Skipping eggs may open your eyes to other more interesting breakfast opportunities, and there is no need for them in baking. (See the recipes starting on page 124 for egg-free breakfast ideas.)

FOODS CONTAINING EGGS TO ELIMINATE

- All egg whites and whole eggs from chickens, ducks, or any other bird.

- Any food containing whole eggs or egg whites, such as mayonnaise, conventional baked goods, and meringue. (Be aware that eggless mayonnaise probably contains inflammatory oils—instead, you could make your own using the recipe on page 230).

■ Look for egg and egg white on all ingredient labels.

EGG-FREE FOODS TO INCORPORATE

■ In baking, any of the following are equivalent to 2 eggs: 1 very ripe banana, well mashed; ¼ cup applesauce or pureed pumpkin; or any egg replacer product (such as Bob's Red Mill or Ener-G) that is gluten-free. (The best grain-free baking flours for you to use are coconut flour and cassava flour.)

■ Try a delicious breakfast hash made with shredded sweet potatoes or shaved Brussels sprouts and onions, fried in ghee or coconut oil until crispy. A tablespoon of nutritional yeast can add an eggy, cheesy effect.

■ Grain- and egg-free toast with avocado slices and sea salt makes an excellent breakfast sandwich replacement. I like delicious cassava-based bread products. You could also add some salmon or a grass-fed beef patty.

■ Black salt contains a sulfur taste that is reminiscent of eggs. Try it in savory breakfast dishes.

■ Try vegetable soup or organic chicken sausage for breakfast.

Day Eight for Elimin8: Nightshades

Nightshades contain alkaloids, which are inflammatory for some people, especially those with rheumatoid arthritis, lupus, and other autoimmune conditions, or those with unexplained joint pain, digestive, or skin problems.[22] Many nightshades are inedible (like morning glories) and many are poisonous (like belladonna). Edible nightshades are some of the most popular foods—like potatoes and tomatoes—and don't bother most people severely.

However, if you have chronic health issues, you may be sensitive to them. We're going to find out if you are.

NIGHTSHADES TO ELIMINATE

- Tomatoes

- Potatoes (all types except sweet potatoes)

- Eggplant

- Peppers, all types, including bell peppers and all hot peppers

- Pimientos

- Tomatillos

- Goji berries

- Cayenne pepper

- Chili powder

- Curry powder

- Paprika

- Red pepper flakes

- Tobacco (Do you need another reason not to smoke? Here's one more.)

NIGHTSHADE SUBSTITUTES TO INCORPORATE

What, no salsa? No tomato sauce? *No French fries?* Fortunately, there are plenty of foods that can stand in for your favorite nightshade foods.

- Sweet potatoes—baked, mashed, dried into chips, or made into fries. I love Japanese sweet potatoes.

- Any root vegetable cut into French-fry shapes, brushed with coconut oil or ghee, and baked until crispy.

- Carrots, beets, pumpkin, or butternut squash cooked until soft and pureed into sauce.

- Make salsa or pico de gallo with chopped cucumbers, chopped jicama or daikon radish, sweet onions, minced fresh garlic, cilantro, and sea salt. Chopped mangoes are also a nice addition.

LOOKING AHEAD

Now that you have fully eliminated everything you will keep out of your life for the next few weeks and you have all the information you need about why each of these foods may be inflammatory to you, how to get them out of your life, and what you get to eat and do instead, you are ready to begin the next phase of your plan. This is the part where you will significantly calm your inflammation and get your body in a state of heightened awareness and increased vitality. You are about to feel better, and fast, so get ready to experience the life you can have when your inflammation subsides.

5

ELIMIN8 OR CORE4: COOL INFLAMMATION AND HEAL

Welcome to the heart and soul of your elimination journey. Ultimately, you are not eliminating certain foods in order to punish yourself with another diet. You are eliminating chronic inflammation. You are eliminating brain fog, fatigue, digestive problems, weight gain, or whatever health issues inflammation is causing in you. You are eliminating the confusion as to what is best for your body and what isn't.

Over the next four or eight weeks, you will form better habits, learn how to eat differently, and enjoy how it feels to reduce inflammation and restore health. I've got lots of tips, treats, and support for you as we walk through these next few weeks together. Fall in love with the process of becoming the best version of yourself. Wellness is sacred art and you are the masterpiece. Each week you will have a list of things to do, a pep talk to keep you going, and a weekly indulgence—something fun and decadent feeling—to anticipate. Here is what you will get in this chapter:

1. Lists of all the amazing, delicious, wholesome, anti-inflammatory foods you *get to eat*. Although your food list on the Core4 track will be longer, you will find that even on the Elimin8 track, you will have an impressively long list of foods to enjoy.

2. A list of the eight inflammatory habits you will also be eliminating—or if they aren't all problems for you, choose the ones that are. You'll be eliminating one each week.

3. Pre-week prep steps, or a list of things to do before each week.

4. Sample meal plans for a week of anti-inflammatory eating for the Core4 and Elimin8 tracks.

5. A week-by-week walk-through with lots of things to learn and do.

....

Seriously, Don't Eat That

Don't go off your plan. That's my initial, strongly worded advice. If you do, you will compromise your anti-inflammatory efforts. Besides, there are so many delicious nutrient-dense foods you *can* eat—why undermine all your hard work and lessen the power of this plan? However, I understand that sometimes it can happen by accident (or "accidentally on purpose"). Here's what to do if you slip up:

- **If it happens in the first two weeks of the Core4 track or in the first four weeks of the Elimin8 track:** Start over. Yep, right back to Day One. Harsh, perhaps, but I mean it. I want you to get the best results and know exactly what your body loves and hates. If you want this program to work, going off your plan means you get booted back to the beginning.

- **If it happens in the second two weeks of the Core4 track or in the second four weeks of the Elimin8 track:** Keep going. You will have compromised the effectiveness of the program somewhat (to a degree equivalent to the extent of what and how much you ate), but by then your inflammation should be down significantly, so you may be able to handle it better.

That said, if you go off your plan once, *don't do it again.* Don't let all your work be for nothing. The final results will be worth the effort to stay with the program exactly as prescribed for you. I don't like the word *cheat.* This is not about all the foods you can't have, the foods that tempt you to cheat. If something potentially causes you inflammation, you want to know for sure whether it works for your body or doesn't work for your body. Forget about dieting, deprivation, shame, and rules and regulations. Focus on loving your body enough to discover the foods that make you feel better, not worse. Stay conscious of this deeper purpose.

WHAT TO EAT

Instead of fixating on the foods you are not eating until reintroduction so that you can wipe the inflammatory slate clean (I've made those foods clear in the previous chapter), let's focus on all the delicious, healing foods that you can eat, no matter which track you're on, by category, including how much of each you should try to fit into your diet every day or week. (Of course, if you know you are allergic to something on this list, cross that off.) Here's what to eat.

Clean Protein

Aim for 1 to 1½ palm-size portions per meal, so your meals always include a protein. And while we are aiming for these portions, not all proteins are created equal. Here I have listed them in order of priority—as much as possible, eat most of your proteins from sources at the top of the list, and eat the least from the protein sources at the bottom.

SEAFOOD

Focus on seafood as your primary source of protein. Unless you are allergic to fish or shellfish, seafood is an excellent source of nutrition and good fats. These are the lower-mercury seafood items that I recommend:

- Alaskan salmon, wild-caught

- Albacore tuna (U.S., Canada, wild, pole-caught)

- Anchovies

- Arctic char

- Atlantic mackerel

- Barramundi

- Bass (saltwater, striped, black)

- Butterfish

- Catfish

- Clam

- Cod (Alaskan)

- Crab (domestic)

- Crawfish/crayfish

- Croaker (Atlantic)

- Flounder

- Herring

- Lobster

- Mahimahi

- Mussels

- Oysters

- Pollock

- Rainbow trout

- Sardines

- Scallops

- Shrimp

- Skipjack tuna (U.S., Canada, wild, pole-caught)

- Sole (Pacific)

- Squid (calamari)

- Tilapia

- Tuna (canned chunk light)

- Whitefish

- Yellowfin tuna (U.S. Atlantic, wild, pole-caught)

- Yellowfin tuna (Western Central Pacific, wild, handline-caught)

ORGANIC POULTRY, PREFERABLY FROM PASTURED OR GAME BIRDS

- Chicken
- Duck
- Goose
- Ostrich
- Quail
- Turkey

ORGANIC MEAT, PREFERABLY FROM GRASS-FED, PASTURED, OR GAME ANIMALS

- Beef
- Bison
- Elk
- Lamb
- Pork
- Rabbit
- Venison

When you are purchasing animal proteins, there are a few key words or descriptions you should look for to help you get the best quality you can to match your budget.

- Seafood should be labeled "wild-caught" and should be on the list of fish lower in mercury. When eating fish like tuna and bass, go for the specific sources I listed and choose brands that have verifiable testing done on mercury levels. There are many conscious brands that go above and beyond to provide safe, healthy low-mercury sources of these fish.

- Beef should be labeled as being from grass-fed, organic cows.

- Poultry and pork are preferably free-range and pasture-raised.

- If buying organic, you can buy a fattier cut of meat on the bone. Organic fats contain wonderful nutrients and minerals.

■ If you can't find organic meats or they do not fit into your budget, choose lean cuts only, as conventionally raised animals can store inflammatory toxins in their fat.

Phasing in Animal Protein

If you haven't been eating meat and have decided to try reintroducing it, start off by bringing meat in slowly to wake up your GI system. Many people who have eaten a vegetarian or vegan diet can suffer from low stomach acid, making it difficult to digest protein. Consider taking digestive enzyme supplements and betaine HCL with pepsin or ox bile before meals to help out your digestion in the beginning until your body adjusts. It *will* adjust.

Plant-Based Protein Sources

If you want to go lighter on the clean animal proteins, bring in more sources of plant-based protein.

CORE4 FRIENDLY

■ Hempeh (tempeh made from hempseed): 22 grams protein per 4 ounces

■ Natto (organic non-GMO): 31 grams protein per 1 cup

■ Tempeh (organic non-GMO): 31 grams protein per 1 cup

■ Hemp protein powder: 12 grams protein per 4 tablespoons

■ Hemp hearts/hempseed: 40 grams protein per 1 cup

■ Sacha inchi seed protein powder: 24 grams protein per ¼ cup

■ Lentils: 18 grams protein per 1 cup

■ Mung beans: 14 grams protein per 1 cup

- Pili nuts: 13 grams protein per 1 cup

- Chickpeas: 15 grams protein per 1 cup

- Almond butter: 6 grams protein per ¼ cup

ELIMIN8 AND CORE4 FRIENDLY

- Maca powder: 3 grams protein per 1 tablespoon

- Peas: 9 grams protein per 1 cup cooked peas (note that fresh legumes in pods are permitted on the Elimin8 track)

- Nutritional yeast: 5 grams protein per 1 tablespoon

- Chlorella or spirulina: 4 grams protein per 1 tablespoon

- Spinach: 3 grams protein per ½ cup cooked spinach

- Avocado: 2 grams protein per ½ avocado

- Broccoli: 2 grams protein per ½ cup cooked broccoli

- Brussels sprouts: 2 grams protein per ½ cup

- Artichokes: 4 grams protein per ½ cup

- Asparagus: 2.9 grams protein per 1 cup

Produce

Vegetables are the key to a nutrient-dense, anti-inflammatory diet, and they should comprise the bulk of yours. See each category below for the amount to include daily.

....

Prioritize Organics

When possible, always choose organic fruits and vegetables. When it's not possible, wash produce thoroughly. Fill sink with cold water and add one cup white vinegar. Allow fruits and vegetables to soak for 15 minutes.

Rinse, pat dry, and store. For more information on the vegetables most tainted with pesticides and those that are less contaminated and okay to buy nonorganic, see the list of the Dirty Dozen and the Clean Fifteen published and updated yearly by the Environmental Working Group.[1]

VEGETABLES

No serving size limit, but aim for at least 4 cups of vegetables a day! Plan on having at least 1-plus cups of vegetables per meal and with your snacks. Focus on getting a variety of different colors, with an emphasis on green leafy vegetables, which contain folate, necessary for supporting methylation pathways. Look at all the different and awesome yummy vegetables you can have! I hope you will explore and try new options. Vegetables should be the core and focus of your diet.

- Artichokes
- Arugula
- Asparagus
- Bok choy
- Broccoli
- Broccoli sprouts
- Brussels sprouts
- Cabbage
- Cauliflower
- Celery
- Chard
- Chives
- Collard greens
- Cucumbers
- Dulse
- Endive
- Ginger
- Jicama
- Kale
- Kelp
- Kohlrabi
- Kombu
- Leeks
- Lettuce

- Mushrooms
- Nori
- Okra
- Olives
- Radishes
- Rhubarb
- Rutabaga
- Scallions
- Seaweed
- Spinach
- Sprouts (alfalfa, bean, broccoli, etc.)
- Squash
- Swiss chard
- Turnips
- Water chestnuts

FRUIT (ESPECIALLY LOW-FRUCTOSE FRUITS)

You can eat any fruit on the Core4 track, and any fruit except goji berries (these are nightshades) on the Elimin8 track. Fruit is nutrient-dense and full of immune-balancing antioxidants, but prioritize fruits with lower fructose for best results, because fructose, in higher amounts, can impact the liver, digestion, and insulin and blood sugar levels. As a general rule, eat more vegetables than fruit. Here are the best fruit choices:

- Avocados
- Bananas
- Blackberries
- Blueberries
- Cantaloupe
- Clementines
- Grapefruit
- Honeydew melon
- Kiwifruit
- Lemons
- Limes
- Oranges
- Muskmelon
- Papayas
- Passion fruit
- Pineapple

- Raspberries
- Rhubarb

- Strawberries
- Tangelos

Healthy Fats

Aim for at least 1 to 3 tablespoons per meal, whether you're cooking, using it as a dressing, or just taking it straight! Focus on having some healthy fat at every meal and snack. Fats have been controversial in the past, but the scientific and nutrition communities are now recognizing how essential they are for health—not at all the disease-promoting substances people once believed they were. Use the recommended fats (but not the inflammatory fats listed on page 98) for cooking, dressing food, adding to smoothies, or eating with a spoon. If you're not used to eating healthy fats from real foods, start off slowly and gradually increase to a healthy amount. Your gallbladder (if you have one), pancreas, and liver probably won't be used to much fat if you've been following a low-fat diet for years, and will need to warm up again.

Fat Myths and Truths

Over the past half a century, there has been an endless barrage of misinformation and propaganda regarding dietary fat. Although old belief systems die hard, we know now that healthy fats do not cause heart disease. Let's bust the fat myths and set the record straight once and for all.

As babies, we were all born relying on fat in the form of breast milk for brain development and energy. The human brain requires a lot of energy to work properly and from a biological and evolutionary perspective, the most sustainable form of energy for optimal brain health is good fat. (I cover this in more detail in my plant-based keto book, *Ketotarian.*) Your brain is composed of 60 percent fat (more than any other organ in your body), and as much as 25 percent of the body's cholesterol is located in the brain. Moreover, we need cholesterol and healthy fat to make healthy hormones and support nerve growth and a healthy immune system. It should be no surprise that some of the many side effects of cholesterol-lowering statin drugs include memory loss, nerve pain, hormonal problems, low sex drive, and erectile dysfunction—the very functions cholesterol and healthy fats support. The healthy fats that we use in Elimin8 are essential for optimal wellness.

COLD-PRESSED OILS, TO ENJOY RAW (DON'T USE THESE FOR COOKING)

- Extra-virgin olive oil

- Extra-virgin avocado oil

- Extra-virgin coconut oil

OILS AND FATS FOR COOKING

- Avocado oil

- Olive oil (not extra virgin)

- Coconut oil

- Grass-fed ghee (clarified butter—this comes from milk, but because the lactose and casein are no longer present, it is fine to eat)

- Palm shortening (organic only)

Herbs

Not only do herbs and spices enhance the flavor of foods, but they add nutrients, and many are highly anti-inflammatory. Enjoy fresh or dried herbs and spices in any amount that tastes good to you.

- Basil
- Bay leaf
- Cilantro
- Dill
- Lavender
- Lemon balm

- Mint
- Oregano
- Parsley
- Rosemary
- Sage

Spices

- Allspice
- Annatto
- Caraway
- Cardamom
- Celery seed
- Cinnamon
- Clove
- Coriander
- Cumin
- Fennel
- Fenugreek
- Garlic
- Ginger

- Horseradish
- Juniper
- Juniper berry
- Mace
- Mustard
- Nutmeg
- Peppercorns (these are not nightshades)
- Sea salt
- Star anise
- Sumac
- Turmeric
- Vanilla bean (organic, no additives)

Beverages

- Water

- Tea (should be organic)

- Coconut water (unsweetened)

- Kombucha (look out for added sugar after fermentation, to make this tart drink sweeter; the tarter it tastes, the better)

- Carbonated water (no added sweeteners)

- Green juices (fresh-pressed green vegetables, lemon, lime, and ginger; be mindful of the sugar content)

- Organic bone broth

For the Core4 Track Folks Only

If you are doing the Core4 track, you do not have to eliminate legumes, nuts and seeds (and their oils and butters), eggs, or nightshades. You can include all of these in your diet, so consider those added to the above food list. However, these next four weeks are a great opportunity to get out of your food rut. Explore the wide world of delicious foods you normally don't eat to nourish your body in a fresh new way.

How to Soak Nuts and Seeds

Core4 people: Activate your nuts! Soaking nuts and seeds will make them more digestible, and their wonderful nutrients will be more usable for your body.

1. Put the nuts or seeds that you want to soak in a bowl and add water to cover.

2. Add 1 to 2 tablespoons of your favorite sea salt.

3. Cover the bowl and let them soak on the counter or in the fridge for about 7 hours, or overnight.

4. Drain the nuts or seeds and rinse to remove the salt. Spread them out on a rack to dehydrate.

5. Dry the nuts or seeds in a dehydrator until they are slightly crispy. If you don't have a dehydrator, you can dry them in the oven at a low temperature until they are slightly crispy. If you choose not to dry them, they typically will last in the fridge for a few days before they begin to become moldy.

If soaking nuts and seeds isn't your thing, there are brands that sell soaked and sprouted nuts and seeds.

CHOOSING YOUR INFLAMMATORY HABIT ELIMINATION LIST

One of the unique features of this individualized plan is that you will be eliminating some inflammatory lifestyle habits. Food is key to an elimination diet, but there are also some potent nonfood factors that can contribute to systemic inflammation and health decline. If you have lifestyle habits that harm your body and brain as well as your emotions and spirit, then even if you do eat everything perfectly during your elimination journey, you are unintentionally sabotaging your healthy efforts. These lifestyle habits can be just as inflammatory as foods, if not more than, so let's get them out of your life!

I believe that breaking the following eight bad habits is crucial to feeling better. You may not have all eight habits right now, but most of us have at least a few. If you are doing the Elimin8 track, you will see one of these habits highlighted during each of the eight weeks. If you are doing the Core4 track, you will be stopping after four weeks, but you can still look ahead to the second four weeks for information on other inflammatory habits you want to work on. Read up on the ones that you would like to change.

Unlike foods you can simply decide not to eat, these habits can be deeply ingrained. I don't expect you to drop them just like that and never look back. This may take some time, but this is your chance to begin phasing them out of your life, so that you can live better, stronger, and with greater happiness and purpose as well as improved health. I also include them to help grow your awareness that it's not just food that can impact your health. You can be eating the perfect, inflammation-calming foods in your plan, but if you are serving yourself a big slice of stress every day, you are unintentionally sabotaging your healthy intentions. Stress and stressful behaviors, as well as a lack of connection to yourself, others, and your life purpose, can all contribute to poor health and inflammation, so working on changing these habits can do a lot to support your process here.

> It's not just food that can impact your health.

These are the inflammatory habits I would like to see you release. Identify the ones that you know are a problem for you and look out for them as we work through the next four or eight weeks. Each week I will feature one of them, with detailed advice about why it is inflammatory and how to give it up, replacing it with better, anti-inflammatory habits. Many people would benefit from doing them all. Here's a preview of the lifestyle habits we'll be targeting:

1. Prolonged sitting (page 131)

2. Staring at screens too much (page 140)

3. Toxin exposure (including molds) (page 149)

4. Negativity (page 158)

5. Monkey mind (racing thoughts) (page 167)

6. Emotional eating (page 174)

7. Social isolation and/or social media addiction (page 182)

8. Lack of higher purpose (page 189)

YOUR ANTI-INFLAMMATORY LIFE BEGINS NOW

Let's begin the four- or eight-week period of your inflammation elimination. As you get started, you may feel some detox-like symptoms, like headaches or changes to your digestion, but these should pass in a few days, and then you should start to feel energized, clearheaded, and fantastic.

Both tracks should begin here. After the pre-planning steps listed on the following pages, move on to Week One. If you are doing the Core4 track, proceed through Week Four, then move on to the next chapter. Elimin8 folks, stay with this process for eight weeks.

SAMPLE MEAL PLANS

These meal plans are only suggestions, using either the Core4 track recipes (starting on page 193) or Elimin8 track recipes (starting on page 219). You could follow your meal plan exactly for the first week, to learn the flow, or you can have the same thing every week over the next four or eight weeks. You could follow it with modifications, or you could ignore it completely and eat what you want, as long as it conforms to your food list and you do not include any of your eliminated foods. This meal plan is for *inspiration*, a means of illustrating how to eat successfully.

In your meal plan, you will get a suggested breakfast, lunch, snack, and dinner that conforms to your Core4 or Elimin8 food list.

Sample Core4 Meal Plan

	BREAKFAST	ELIXIR
MONDAY	Coconut–Butternut Squash Porridge (page 193)	Tropical Spice Juice (page 246)
TUESDAY	Hummus and Greens Breakfast Bowl (page 194)	Anti-Inflammatory Turmeric Milk (Golden Milk) (page 251)
WEDNESDAY	Spiced Mushroom and Veggie Hash with Sunshine Eggs (page 197)	Beautifying Blue-Green Mermaid Latte (page 251)
THURSDAY	Sweet Potato Breakfast Skillet (page 198)	Blueberry Blast Juice (page 247)
FRIDAY	Nuts, Seeds, and Coconut Granola (page 196)	Dr. Will Cole's Gut-Healing Smoo (page 249)
SATURDAY	Mexican Avocado Baked Eggs (page 195)	Refreshing Adrenal-Balancing Iced Tea (page 248)
SUNDAY	Fluffy Grain-Free Pancakes (page 193)	Treg Pumper-Upper Smoothie (page 250)

LUNCH	SNACK	DINNER
Quick Dal with Cauliflower Rice (page 202)	Chocolate, Coconut, and Hemp Energy Balls (page 215)	Pesto-Stuffed Chicken Breasts with Chunky Tomato Sauce (page 209)
Smoked Salmon Salad (page 203)	Crunchy Roasted Chickpeas (page 216)	Weeknight Beef Pho (page 212)
Garlicky Butternut Squash Noodles with Kielbasa (page 199)	Zucchini Hummus Cucumber Sushi Rolls (page 218)	Root Vegetable Curry (page 211)
Mango Tuna Salad–Stuffed Popovers (page 201)	Chili-Spiced Nuts and Cranberries (page 215)	Cauliflower-Walnut Tacos (page 206)
Chopped Kale Salad with Thai Peanut Dressing (page 199)	Cauliflower-Nut Flatbread (page 214)	Pan-Seared Salmon on Bitter Greens with Sweet Cherries (page 208)
Waldorf Salad Wrap (page 204)	Guacamole-Stuffed Baby Bells (page 217)	Ginger-Garlic Shrimp and Cabbage (page 207)
Sweet Potato BLTs (page 203)	Buffalo Chicken Dip (page 213)	Breakfast-Anytime Nachos (page 205)

Sample Elimin8 Meal Plan

	BREAKFAST	ELIXIR
MONDAY	Power Greens Smoothie (page 222)	The Green Queen Juice (page 247)
TUESDAY	Brussels Sprouts, Bacon, Apple, and Salmon Skillet (page 220)	Anti-Inflammatory Turmeric Milk (Golden Milk) (page 251)
WEDNESDAY	Sweet Potato–Date Smoothie (page 225)	Beautifying Blue-Green Mermaid Latte (page 251)
THURSDAY	Breakfast Steaks with Sweet Potato Hash Browns (page 219)	Thyroid-Boosting Smoothie (page 2
FRIDAY	Shrimp, Bacon, and Okra with Garlicky Cauliflower Grits (page 224)	Dr. Will Cole's Gut-Healing Smoot (page 249)
SATURDAY	Herb-Crushed Cauliflower Steaks with Mushroom-Onion Scramble (page 221)	Rejuvenating Celery Juice (page 24
SUNDAY	Sausage-Stuffed Apples (page 222)	Treg Pumper-Upper Smoothie (page 250)

LUNCH	SNACK	DINNER
Lemony Fish Soup with Herbs and Greens (page 227)	Crunchy Veggie Rolls with Homemade Ranch Dressing (page 240)	Chicken and Vegetable Lo Mein (page 233)
Chicken Zoodle Soup (page 227)	Dilled Smoked Salmon–Cucumber Bites (prep the night before and chill overnight) (page 241)	Creamy Coconut-Ginger Squash Soup (page 235)
Shrimp Cakes with Creamy Dilled Slaw (page 229)	Prosciutto Chips, Three Ways (page 244)	Roasted Pork Chops with Olives and Grapes (page 238)
Cauliflower-Broccoli Tabbouleh (page 226)	Quick Veggie Pickles (make the day before—has to chill 24 hours) (page 244)	Buttery Garlic-Tarragon Pan-Seared Scallops with Shaved Asparagus Salad (page 232)
Steak and Carrot Noodle Bowl with Chimichurri Sauce (page 230)	Fig and Olive Tapenade (page 242)	Jicama Fish Tacos (page 236)
Veggie-Avocado Mash Coconut Wraps (page 232)	Snack-Size Italian Meatballs (prep the night before, cook the day of) (page 245)	Pan-Seared Flounder with Kohlrabi, Carrot, and Apple Slaw (page 237)
Salmon, Beets, and Shaved Fennel Salad (page 228)	Lemon-Thyme Parsnip Fries (page 243)	Spiced Beef Burgers with Sweet-and-Sour Red Cabbage (page 239)

Also keep in mind that you Core4 people can use the Elimin8 recipes as well. You will also get a special medicinal elixir to have in the midmorning. I have developed these various juices, smoothies, teas, and tonics specifically for their anti-inflammatory action, but they also contain medicinal ingredients (like adaptogenic herbs or superfoods), so you can switch these out in whichever way you like or browse the recipes starting on page 246. Some of these elixirs also target particular systems like the adrenals, thyroid, or skin, but they are all appropriate for everyone, no matter what track you are on or which area you have the most inflammation.

PRE-WEEK PREP STEPS

Do these eight things before starting each week:

1. Consult the meal plans and the recipes beginning on page 122 for some inspiration.

2. Choose the meals you want to make this week. If you aren't sure if a food you want to eat is allowed, review the food lists at the beginning of this chapter, beginning on page 108.

3. Fill out the blank meal plan with your food choices for the week.

4. Go grocery shopping to get everything you need for the week.

5. Check out the featured inflammatory habit of the week and decide if this is something you need to give up.

6. Consult your toolbox (beginning on page 65) and decide which tools you want to use this week.

7. Get in the right mindset. Tell yourself you are ready and you can do this!

8. Repeat this prep before each new week.

WEEK ONE

■ Before you begin, do your pre-week prep steps (page 126).

Your Typical Day

- As soon as you wake up, sit quietly for a few minutes, breathing deeply and thinking about your mantra (from your toolbox, beginning on page 65). Prepare for your day. This is also a good time to meditate for 10 or 15 minutes, if you can. Let's kick this off right.

- Eat your planned breakfast, and if you are leaving for the day, pack up your lunch and a snack so you don't get caught hungry and tempted to stray from your plan.

- Choose at least one tool from your toolbox (starting on page 65) to include today.

- Eat your planned lunch, snack, and dinner, focusing on the novelty and excitement of new foods and the vibrant health that will soon be yours!

- Try to get moving for about 30 minutes on most days of the week, whether that is structured exercise or walking. Your goal is to sweat when you exercise, but if you aren't used to exercising, start small and work up to that goal.

- Do one of the replacement behaviors for the inflammatory habit you are working on this week.

- Before bed, repeat your mantra and think about your day. If you feel like you want it or need it, this is also a good time to meditate for 10 or 15 minutes.

WEEK ONE MEAL PLAN

	BREAKFAST	ELIXIR
MONDAY		
TUESDAY		
WEDNESDAY		
THURSDAY		
FRIDAY		
SATURDAY		
SUNDAY		

LUNCH	SNACK	DINNER

Your Weekly Pep Talk

You are probably pretty motivated this week. Most people are when they first get started. You might also be a little nervous. Can you do it? Will you succeed? Of course you can, and of course you will! This elimination program might be much different from diets you've tried before. While weight loss may have been your focus in the past, this time, weight loss (if you need it) is a perk on this plan. The focus here is to learn what foods are good for you and what foods cause inflammation in you, and this is how you get there. This is how you will grow healthier, stronger, and more energized.

You are rebooting your body so that it can start working better and giving you better feedback about how it reacts to what you eat and how you live. This week is an opportunity to begin listening. Pay attention to how you feel each day this week—after you eat something, after you exercise, after you spend time outside or with the people you love. Let your body speak to you. Open that door. This is the beginning of a beautiful friendship. There is a learning curve here, and each week will feel easier and more natural, so don't get discouraged if this feels difficult at first. As with anything new and good that you do for yourself, even when it feels foreign or a little uncomfortable, remind yourself that what you are doing will make your health and your life better, for you and for everyone who depends on you and loves you.

> **You are rebooting your body.**

Indulge Yourself: Forest Bathing

This week I want you to do something special for yourself: Take a walk through a wooded area. You can do this in any season—dress appropriately, of course. Walking in the woods (or a forest) has proven benefits. The Japanese call it *shinrin-yoku*, or "forest bathing," and studies show that it not only reduces feelings of stress and anxiety and increases feelings of energy, it boosts natural killer cells in the body, a sign that the immune system is invigorated. One theory is that the essential oils from trees cause this immune boost. This indulgence will relax you and get you more in touch with your own natural rhythms. If you like to walk alone and can do so safely, then great. Or bring a dog or a friend. If you choose to walk with someone else, try not to talk too much. Treat this like a walking meditation. Breathe deeply and focus on the beauty all around you—the colors, the shapes, the feel of the air, the texture of the trees, the wildlife. Let nature work its magic on you.

Inflammatory Habit 1: Prolonged Sitting

Human bodies aren't meant to sit all day. They are meant to walk, run, lift, carry, even swim. Squatting or even sitting on the ground is better for your body than sitting in a chair. Obviously you have to sit some of the time, but let's cut that time way down, starting now. You'll feel the difference right away.

WHY GIVE IT UP (FOR NOW): You may have heard that "sitting is the new smoking." That may be a slight overstatement, but there is no question sitting is bad for your health. When you sit, your muscles relax and your blood doesn't pump as efficiently. That means less blood to your heart, higher blood pressure, and less efficient elimination of fat and waste products. Prolonged sitting has been linked to insulin resistance; a higher risk of cancers, including colon and breast cancer; muscle atrophy; circulation problems; neck and back strain; and even premature death.[2] Bonus: You burn 30 percent more calories standing than sitting, so if you sit less, you will probably drop some weight, even without changing anything else.

HOW TO GIVE IT UP: Try these tips for phasing out sitting in favor of more activity.

- **Remind yourself.** When you are sitting for a long time, whether at a desk, in a car, or in front of the television, set a reminder on your watch, phone, or computer to get up and walk around for five to ten minutes every hour. Don't think you will get less work done—the stimulation will help you work more efficiently, which should more than make up for the time *not* sitting.

- **Stand up.** At work, invest in a standing desk (or make one with things you already have), so that you spend some of your day on your feet. Some companies will pay for these desks for their employees.

- **Multitask.** If you are watching television at home, find things to do that keep you moving, like folding laundry, doing sit-ups and leg lifts or basic yoga poses, or decluttering something. At least get up and walk around during commercials instead of fast-forwarding past them.

- **Take travel breaks.** When driving long distances, try to stop for at least a few minutes every hour. On a train or airplane, get up and walk around or at least stand and stretch hourly.

WHAT TO DO INSTEAD: Never sit when you can stand; never stand when you can walk. The more activity you incorporate into your day, the less time you will have for sitting. Sometimes you have to sit, of course, but when it's not essential, challenge yourself to stand up and/or move around.

ACTIVITIES TO INCORPORATE: The more you move in natural ways throughout your day, the better your body and mind will work. If you like going to the gym, maybe get back in the habit, but if gyms aren't for you, that's fine, too. A daily walk can make a big difference.

- **Walking** is one of the best things you can do for your body. You are built to walk. Take a walk around the block or through the park, or go on a hike. If the weather is cold or wet, you could walk indoors, through a mall, the grocery store, or a museum. Meet a friend for a walk instead of coffee or lunch (or bring your coffee along). You don't have to walk fast. Move your body and encourage circulation at a level that feels doable for you. If the impact is a problem, try walking in a swimming pool.

- **Pets** offer a good opportunity for walking. Walk your dog, or if you're a cat person, try walking your cat.

- **Go on a bike ride** or take a spin class.

- **Play an active game with kids**—Twister, anyone? Capture the flag? Tag, you're it?

- **Join a sports team or take lessons** in tennis, golf, jiu jitsu, pickleball (it's a thing), or another sport you've always wanted to learn.

- **Train for a charity walk, a 5K, a triathlon, or any other competitive activity.** You don't have to be an athlete—there are events like these for most fitness levels.

HOW DO YOU FEEL AFTER WEEK ONE? Notice if you feel differently, if you are having detox symptoms, or if any of your previous symptoms are starting to resolve.

_____

_____

_____

_____

WEEK TWO

■ Before you begin, do your pre-week prep steps (page 126).

Your Typical Day

- As soon as you wake up, sit quietly for a few minutes, breathing deeply and thinking about the mantra from your toolbox (starting on page 65). Prepare for your day. This is also a good time to meditate for 10 or 15 minutes. It takes a few weeks to make a habit, so this morning ritual won't be a habit yet, but it should begin to feel more natural.

- Eat your planned breakfast. Pack up your lunch and snack. Be sure to keep your kitchen stocked with allowed foods and keep the eliminated foods out of your line of sight.

- Pick at least one tool from your toolbox (starting on page 65) to include today. The more consistently you use these tools, the more quickly and effectively you will reduce your inflammation and symptoms.

- Eat your planned lunch, snack, and dinner. Enjoy your food!

- Try to get moving for about 30 minutes on most days of the week, whether that is structured exercise or walking. If you want to exercise longer, that's fine, too. Cardio activities and weight lifting are both great for generating BDNF (brain-derived neurotrophic factor), which helps to reduce inflammation and strengthen neural pathways.

- Do one of the replacement behaviors for the inflammatory habit you are working on this week. That habit will get a little bit easier to avoid every day you resist it.

- Before bed, repeat your mantra and think about your day. If you feel like you want it or need it, this is also a good time to meditate for 10 or 15 minutes. You may discover you sleep better with this nightly ritual.

Your Weekly Pep Talk

This week, you may feel proud of yourself for getting through the first week, but you may also start to have more cravings or be tempted to go off plan. Although it's only Week Two, it can feel like you've gone *forever* without your favorite thing, whether that's cheese or chocolate or staring at a screen. This is a temporary obstacle and it will pass. Remember that if you go off plan, you will have to start over. No sense in wasting that first week you've already done! Next week, all of this will seem even easier and more natural, so stay strong.

To help you get through this week, try doing something spiritual. A few studies have supported the idea that those who have a regular spiritual practice tend to live longer. The reason may be interleukin 6 (IL-6). Increased levels are associated with increased disease, and one study showed that those who attend church were half as likely to have elevated IL-6.[3] This may be because of the social support people receive from their spiritual community, but there may be other factors. Another study shows that those who have a sense of spiritual well-being had a better quality of life, even when they had chronic pain—many spiritual people use prayer for pain management.[4] There are other studies that have examined the benefits of a spiritual practice for recovery from illness. Anything that gives your life greater meaning has been demonstrated to have a positive impact on your physical and emotional health, so any spiritual effort on your part will help you to focus less on the daily grind and more on your own higher purpose, whatever that means for you.

WEEK TWO MEAL PLAN

	BREAKFAST	ELIXIR
MONDAY		
TUESDAY		
WEDNESDAY		
THURSDAY		
FRIDAY		
SATURDAY		
SUNDAY		

LUNCH	SNACK	DINNER

If you have a faith you practice, do something extra that's in line with your beliefs. That may mean spending time every morning and/or evening praying (it's fine to do this instead of meditating—both are anti-inflammatory practices) or practicing another ritual that makes you feel connected to something bigger than yourself—even gentle yoga. If you aren't religious, you can still benefit. Bring a new ritual into your life that makes you feel connected to your own higher purpose, your sense of a higher power, or a basic reverence for life. Here are some ideas:

- **Get spiritual.** Visit different religious institutions to see what they are about. Maybe something will strike a chord in you. You might be interested in worshiping every Saturday or Sunday or checking out a meditation center. Getting out into nature can also be a powerful spiritual experience. You don't have to be a member of a particular religion to have a spiritual experience.

- **Zen out.** If you haven't been meditating every morning and/or evening, try doing that this week. See how it feels. Or use that time to pray. You don't have to have any specific beliefs or necessarily feel like you know or understand the nature of a higher power to try reaching out.

- **Brew your potion.** If you are looking for something a little less overtly spiritual, make it a morning ritual to prepare the optional midmorning elixir or therapeutic drink in your meal plan with quiet mindfulness. Drink it slowly, paying attention to everything about the experience. If you need to hang a DO NOT DISTURB sign on your bedroom door and sip it in there, then go for it. (See page 246 for elixir recipes.)

- **Diffuse oil.** Take five minutes to sit near an essential oil diffuser or to sniff an essential oil that makes you feel grounded and centered. Citrus blends and bergamot reduce stress levels, but you may have other favorites. Clary sage is good for hormonal mood swings. Frankincense, cedarwood, and rose are good oils for meditation or spiritual contemplation.

- **Make an altar.** Find a small area, such as a shelf, a small desk or table, or a corner of a room. Cover the area with a scarf, shawl, or other fabric that feels special to you, and decorate it with items that are meaningful to you—mementos, photos, crystals, candles, flowers, or anything else that makes you feel connected to the good things in your life or gives you a sense of calm and well-being. Spend a few minutes each day sitting quietly in front of your altar, contemplating the items there and what they represent in your life.

- **Try earthing.** Take five minutes out of your day to stop what you are doing, take off your shoes, and walk in the grass, sand, or dirt. This is called *earthing*, and it has been shown to calm the mind and body, possibly because of the direct physical contact with the electrons on the surface of the earth.[5] Scientists have studied this! Electrons aside, this direct contact with the planet can feel like a spiritual experience and help us all remember where we came from.

- **Volunteer.** For some people, the most spiritual thing they can do—what provides the greatest sense of a higher purpose—is to help others. Studies show that volunteering can make you live longer, have better health, and increase life satisfaction.[6] What you do could be as simple as petting cats at a shelter or reading to elementary school students, or as complex as laying the groundwork for a new career. It doesn't have to be official volunteering, either. It could mean visiting an elderly neighbor or relative, bringing food to a family experiencing difficulty, or donating to your local food pantry.

Indulge Yourself: Get a Massage

Massages feel like a luxury, but they are essential, especially if you have issues with joints, muscles, and connective tissue, but also if you are working on detoxifying. Massage relaxes tight muscles, calms the mind, and increases circulation, helping boost the activity of a sluggish lymphatic system for more potent waste removal.

As you reduce your levels of inflammation, your body will begin detoxing more rapidly, and massage supports this process. If you have a regular massage therapist, be sure to schedule something during this week. If not, look for deals in your area, such as massages offered free or at reduced cost to get you to try a new therapist or spa, or less expensive massages by massage therapists in training. Or have a loved one give you a massage. The massage doesn't have to be hard or painful, unless you like deep-tissue work. Even gentle stroking along your back, arms, and legs will increase your circulation and help your process. If you can convince someone to give you a massage every day this week (or forever?), even better.

Inflammatory Habit 2: Screen Staring

This one is difficult for those who spend a lot of time on their smartphones, tablets, or computers; who watch a lot of television; or who are avid gamers. The world doesn't make it any easier, with televisions in almost every restaurant and in many other public places, from gyms to doctors' offices to grocery stores. According to recent estimates, American adults spend an average of over ten hours every day staring at screens![7] This addiction is hurting us, reducing our concentration and possibly even rewiring the brains of our children. Start today by monitoring and regulating screen time for you *and* your kids.

WHY GIVE IT UP (FOR NOW): Unfortunately, screen addiction is a real thing—both pervasive and potentially brain-damaging. Several studies have demonstrated actual brain atrophy in those who are addicted to the Internet or gaming, particularly in the brain areas for impulse control, sensitivity to loss, and the ability to have empathy for others.[8] Screen addiction may also compromise the areas that control brain-body communication and has been associated with brain changes similar to those in people with drug addiction.[9] Excessive television watching is linked with the same health issues as too much sitting—an increased risk of diabetes, heart disease, and premature death.[10] There is also something called computer vision syndrome, which can result in eye irritation and eyestrain,[11] vision impairment in children,[12] and even orthopedic issues, with actual names like *text neck* and *cellphone elbow*.[13] Yeah, we have a problem.

It makes sense—think of how differently you use your brain and body when you are interacting directly with the world, compared to when you are staring at a screen. Staring at a screen is either passive or interactive but without the pressures and necessities of face-to-face communication, or even the brainpower it takes to read an actual book. Plus, screens tend to offer bytes of information without requiring sustained concentration. They have light, they have sound, they have flashy colors—they are easy to pay attention to, compared to text on boring old pieces of paper or the conversation of others. We skim through superficial information without spending much time focused on any one subject; some research shows that we may be rewiring our brains to make concentration, attention, and focus more difficult.[14] We could eventually lose these abilities—even lower our capacity for deep and intelligent thought. Yikes. What's the answer? Step away from the screen.

HOW TO GIVE IT UP: Are you already thinking up excuses? Like how you have to work on a computer, or you keep in touch with your kids on your smartphone because they answer only to text messages? Or how you can't miss your favorite show? You aren't going to eliminate screens 100 percent, so don't pawn your TV or resign from your office job just yet. I can guarantee you will feel better if you start regulating and limiting excessive screen staring without compromising the activities that are necessary and that provide you with real pleasure. Today, see if you can cut down your time a little bit:

- After you are done working, resist the urge to surf the Internet. Turn off the screen and do something else.

- Notice how often you check your emails. Can you reduce the time you spend on this, or do it in chunks a few times a day instead of immediately responding to every text or email alert?

- Challenge yourself and your family to find something different to do tonight, other than watching TV or playing video games— something that doesn't involve a screen at all. Can you go out to a (screenless) restaurant? Play a game? Take a walk or a bike ride together? Invite people over? Can you all leave your phones at home? Radical idea, I know, but *I know firsthand that it is possible!* I have worked very hard to incorporate screenless time in my life so I can focus on my family more fully.

This may be difficult today, but as you keep working at chipping away at your screen time, you will feel the difference. My patients report a deep sense of well-being as they wean themselves from screens and start looking more directly and more often at the world and the actual people immediately around them.

WHAT TO DO INSTEAD: You may be a bit rusty, but today is a chance to expand your skill at interacting directly with the world. Look at the people and things and places in your life, not at your electronic devices.

ACTIVITIES TO INCORPORATE: Fresh out of ideas that aren't screen-centric? Try these:

- **Spend time in nature.** There is nothing more healing to the eyes, the brain, and the body than time passed in the natural world. Take a walk in a park, go on a hike, or take a day-trip to a natural area today. If you can't leave your phone at home, at least stash it in the glove box or put it in your purse or pocket and resist the urge to keep taking it out and looking at it.

- **Interact with those in front of you.** Talk directly to your kids. Meet a friend for coffee and keep your phone put away. Walk over to people in your office and tell them what you need to tell them, without defaulting to text or email. Look others directly in the eyes and smile. Notice their reactions. It might feel weird, but the more you do it, the more natural it will be. (Imagine . . . everybody used to do this *all the time*.)

- **Go to the theater or attend a live event or a concert.** Watching a play or a concert, as opposed to watching a movie or a music video, feels completely different. At first you may even find it strenuous, but it is good for your brain. What can you see *live* tonight? Bonus points if it is outdoors and you don't take a video of it with your phone or post anything about it on social media.

- **Take a walk** around your neighborhood, or even indoors somewhere, tuning in to all your senses. What do you see, hear, smell, feel? Notice if you have the impulse to look something up or post about something on social media and try to ride out the impulse.

- **Eat an entire meal without looking at a screen**—no TV, no phone. Pay attention to your food and the company instead. You will eat less and make better food choices when you pay attention to your food.

HOW DO YOU FEEL AFTER WEEK TWO? Describe how you are progressing. Are you starting to feel better? Still having some detox symptoms? What has changed?

_____

_____

_____

_____

_____

WEEK THREE

■ Before you begin, do your pre-week prep steps (page 126).

Your Typical Day

- Are you in the habit of a morning meditation yet? Even sitting quietly and breathing for 5 minutes is powerful. Don't forget to repeat your mantra today.

- Eat your planned breakfast and pack up your lunch and a snack. If you like to eat the same thing every day, that's perfectly fine, as long as it is compliant.

- This week try to include at least two tools from your toolbox, or one more than you were doing last week. Some people find that it is easier to do these on the weekends, when they have a little more time, but do what works in your schedule. The more of these you use, the more your inflammation will respond.

- Eat your planned lunch, snack, and dinner. Are you getting used to new foods yet? Focus on that, not on what you might be "missing" (remember, those are the things that were making you feel not so great!).

- See if you can sweat for 30 minutes for six out of seven days this week. This is a powerful way to reduce inflammation, boost your mood, and keep your motivation high. It's also good for your muscles, joints, digestion, detoxification, blood sugar levels, and immune system.

- Do one of the replacement behaviors for the inflammatory habit you are working on this week. It's okay if it is always the same, or if you do a different one every day.

- Before bed, repeat your mantra and think about your day. Use your mantra to meditate each evening for 10 or 15 minutes.

Repeat it quietly in your mind at a relaxed pace. If you get distracted, bring your focus back to your mantra, without judgment.

Your Weekly Pep Talk

Let's talk about weight. You may have lost some weight by now, if you have weight to lose. If you have been weighing yourself regularly, I would like you to stop doing that this week. Your focus right now is on reducing inflammation and getting healthy. Weight loss is a natural by-product of this process, but weighing yourself daily or even weekly can keep you too focused on that one goal at the expense of a broader view of your health and well-being. I find that once my patients see that they are losing weight, they begin to change their plan in subtle ways to try to lose even more weight. They cut back on food, they overexercise to the point of stress, and they begin to increase inflammation again. This is not the goal right now. The goal is to reduce inflammation so that you can determine your food intolerances and sensitivities. That is job one, and altering the plan compromises this goal.

Set yourself free from the burden of focusing on your weight and focus on how you feel—how the foods you eat and the things you do and even the way you think influence you—physically, emotionally, and spiritually. Let go of the notion that you "should" weigh some particular number and let your spirit soar. Raise your vibration. Make this about your whole being. When you are tempted to step on the scale, breathe and trust yourself. You can weigh yourself at the end of your four or eight weeks if you must, but for now, put the scale away.

WEEK THREE MEAL PLAN

	BREAKFAST	ELIXIR
MONDAY		
TUESDAY		
WEDNESDAY		
THURSDAY		
FRIDAY		
SATURDAY		
SUNDAY		

LUNCH	SNACK	DINNER

Indulge Yourself: Legs-up-the-Wall Pose

This week I want you to try one of the simplest and most restorative yoga asanas I know: Legs-up-the-Wall Pose (technically, this is called Viparita Karani, which means "reversed action"). Metaphorically, I like this pose because much of what we are doing on this elimination journey is reversing the actions that created inflammation and health issues. Physically, this pose is an inversion that almost anyone can do. It is incredibly relaxing and has some profound stress-relieving and circulation-stimulating benefits for those who do it regularly. Here's how to do it:

1. Grab a yoga mat if you have one (or a blanket) and three pillows. Optional items are an eye pillow or a sleep mask, a yoga belt or scarf to keep your legs from sliding apart, and a timer (such as the one on your phone).

2. Put the short end of the yoga mat or a blanket against the wall, so it lies perpendicular to the wall. Put a pillow approximately where your head would be, and two pillows against the wall.

3. Position yourself on the floor next to the wall, with the wall to your side. Slowly lie down on the mat or blanket as you extend your legs up the wall, scooching your hips as close to the wall as you can. Arrange the pillows under you for support in a way that's comfortable. Some people like a pillow under their hips, or one under their shoulders or elbows. You should be lying in an L-shape, with your torso on the ground and your legs straight up, resting on the wall. Your feet can be close together or up to about a foot apart. If you have trouble keeping your legs from falling apart into the splits, wrap your yoga belt or a scarf around your thighs and tie your legs together. You should be able to relax your legs completely. If your knees hyperextend, you could also stuff a pillow behind them, against the wall.

4. Put an eye pillow or sleep mask over your eyes, if that makes it easier for you to keep your eyes closed.

5. Set a timer for 10 or 15 minutes, or if you aren't on a schedule, don't worry about the time. Close your eyes, open your arms out to the sides, palms facing up, and concentrate on relaxing all parts of your body. Breathe slowly and deeply.

6. When you are finished, slowly bend your knees and roll to one side, then scoot away from the wall. Notice how you feel.

7. Repeat daily this week, and whenever you need to restore your energy and focus.

Inflammatory Habit 3: Toxin Exposure

We live in a chemical world, and unfortunately we all have xenobiotics, or substances foreign to the human body, inside of us. Even newborn infants can have industrial chemicals and pollutants in their umbilical cord blood.[15] The good news is, there are many ways we can get chemicals out of our lives. We can't eliminate them all, but there are ways to reduce exposure to put less of a burden on your body's elimination systems.

WHY GIVE IT UP (FOR NOW): "Giving up" chemical pollutants and biotoxins doesn't seem like such a sacrifice—of course you don't want those poisons in your body. A lot of the things people like to do—for example, wash their hair, wear makeup, clean their houses, keep pests off their lawns, cook on nonstick cookware, and drink from plastic bottles—can involve at least some degree of toxic exposure. Many of those pollutants are potent endocrine disrupters, substances that alter your natural hormone system. Many are carcinogens or neurotoxins or both.

HOW TO GIVE IT UP: Give your body a break and choose natural botanical products and nontoxic cleaners. Detoxifying is about changing some of the products you use and the things you do, and that takes more than a shopping trip. It also takes a change in attitude. Think about all the things you do in your life that contribute to your own toxic burden, then consider how you might change them. Do you have to use nonstick cookware? Have you tried cooking with cast iron or stainless steel and a quality avocado or coconut oil? What about your personal care products and makeup? Think about how devoted you are to particular brands, and how willing you might be to switch to something more natural.

What about indoor air quality? Do you need to douse everything with air freshener? Do you need to sanitize every surface with hard-core chemicals? And what about over-the-counter medications? Do you need that ibuprofen? Do you have to have the allergy medicine or the acid blocker? (Many of these may become unnecessary anyway, as your body cleans itself out and inflammation goes down.)

Also think about convenience versus health. If there are a few things you aren't willing to change—your deal-breakers—then don't change those things. Maybe you are not giving up your favorite hand cream or sauté pan. Okay, but what about all the items you don't really care all that much about, when you think about it? Like that cheap cookware set that is already losing its coating, or the chemicals that make you nervous when you use them on the kitchen counter, or the fancy lipstick that doesn't stay on anyway? You might find you aren't as attached to some of those toxic habits as you thought you were. Bountiful natural alternatives await you.

WHAT TO DO INSTEAD: Popular demand has resulted in many natural products for purchase and lots of readily available information about how to make natural products at home from basic ingredients. Here are some ideas for detoxifying your environment today.

- **Coconut oil** is one of the best substances for personal hygiene. If you have ninety-nine problems, coconut oil can solve about seventy-two of them. Use it to wash your face, brush your teeth, moisturize your skin, and condition your hair (but rinse well, unless you're into the greasy look).

- **Natural beauty products** and makeup are widely available. Look for those that are gluten-free and contain all-natural plant-based ingredients.

- **Clean your home with simple ingredients** you probably already have in your kitchen, like vinegar water spray, baking soda for scrubbing, rubbing alcohol and water for polishing glass and mirrors, and olive or coconut oil for cleaning wood. Or buy natural cleaning products, which are now widely available and getting more affordable all the time as more and more people demand them.

- **Houseplants.** If you can keep them healthy and bug-free, put some houseplants around. They naturally clean the air. An air cleaner in the bedroom is also a good idea, especially if you have pets. You spend a lot of time sleeping, so if the bedroom air is cleaner, you will be, too.

- **Don't use chemical air fresheners.** Essential oil diffusers are a less harmful way to keep your home smelling sweet.

- **Open the windows** (unless you have pollen allergies and it's that season) to freshen and move your indoor air, weather permitting.

- **Decorate with natural materials.** When you replace furniture or decor in your home, seek out materials like hardwood, bamboo, stone, wool, and organic cotton. More processed materials off-gas chemicals into your air.

- **Use a HEPA filter** in your vacuum cleaner and furnace. Consider having your home tested for mold, as this can slow down your healing journey.

- **Use natural products outside.** Many lawn care, garden, and pest control companies now use environmentally friendly and nontoxic products rather than toxic chemicals.

- **Try turmeric.** Medications use up a lot of time in your liver, as your body seeks to process and eliminate their toxic elements. If you have a headache or menstrual pain, try skipping the ibuprofen or acetaminophen and use the spice turmeric as a potent natural anti-inflammatory remedy instead.[16] You can buy it in capsules or find it in the spice aisle, to use in cooking.

- **Sip raw apple cider vinegar.** It sounds counterintuitive, but if you have heartburn or reflux, instead of automatically popping an antacid or a proton pump inhibitor, try a spoonful of this tart treat. Seriously—this is surprisingly effective.

HOW DO YOU FEEL AFTER WEEK THREE? If you haven't noticed much difference before, I bet you are noticing some changes this week. Detoxing may be over by now and you are probably feeling at least some symptom relief as well as seeing some weight loss. Remember, though, that we all respond at our own pace. How is it going for you?

_____

_____

_____

_____

_____

WEEK FOUR

■ Before you begin, do your pre-week prep steps (page 126).

Your Typical Day

- This week, see if you can increase your morning meditation, prayer, or quiet time by 5 minutes. The real power behind this practice is in doing it regularly—every day, day after day. Some people meditate for an hour twice a day, but most of us don't have that kind of time—but that 15 minutes you would have spent mindlessly googling things or watching TV? Give it a try. Don't forget to repeat your mantra today. It can be a part of your meditation, but it doesn't have to be. Also think about it throughout the day.

- Eat your planned breakfast and pack up your lunch and a snack. Stay the course—you are making real progress!

- This week, again, keep going with at least two tools from your toolbox. You may have favorites, and that's great, but see if you can add something new, too.

- Eat your planned lunch, snack, and dinner. Have you found some favorites in the recipes that you like to eat each week? Have you created some new dishes based on the food list? Try to get creative this week with a new recipe, or follow the meal plan exactly, if you haven't yet. Goals like these can help keep you more interested in your meals.

- Keep exercising this week. Like meditation, exercise is most powerful when you do it regularly. Thirty minutes six days a week is ideal. This is powerful, essential self-care that will keep you going, so don't be tempted to think you don't have time for it. It's like brushing your teeth. When you feel like you must do it, like it's not even optional, that's when you know you have succeeded.

WEEK FOUR MEAL PLAN

	BREAKFAST	ELIXIR
MONDAY		
TUESDAY		
WEDNESDAY		
THURSDAY		
FRIDAY		
SATURDAY		
SUNDAY		

LUNCH	SNACK	DINNER

- Are you so over your inflammatory habits? Congratulations! But for many, these will still be difficult. Keep working on the one you have chosen for this week. Remember that even if something feels good in the moment, it's not worth the price if it hurts you in the long run.

- Before bed, repeat your mantra and think about your day. You don't need to meditate with your mantra unless you'd like to, but remember it and reflect on how it may be influencing your subconscious mind to stay true to your goals. Before-bed meditation is also a powerful sleep inducer.

YOUR WEEKLY PEP TALK

Hey, Core4 people, you are on the homestretch! This is your last week, and you have rocked it! But don't give up just yet. You want to take advantage of the entire four weeks to really kick that inflammation to the curb.

If you are on the Elimin8 track, at the end of the week, you will be halfway there—how time flies! Keep going strong—you are doing great!

Chances are good that this week, whether you are doing Core4 or Elimin8, you are feeling pretty good about yourself and experiencing noticeable symptom relief because your inflammation has likely calmed down significantly. However, if you have been doing the Core4 track *and you are not experiencing symptom relief or feeling better,* you may need a stronger intervention. Consider switching to the Elimin8 track and keep going. You may feel more capable of doing more and going longer by now, so join the Elimin8 clan for the final four. Eight weeks might be what it takes to make a real difference in your health. Also, the best way to test the foods you have given up is to make sure your inflammation is way down, so sticking with it longer will give you an even clearer picture of what your body loves best.

This week, pay special attention to any changes in your body. Is your stomach flatter? Do your legs look thinner? Are your arms less jiggly? Are you gaining muscle? Are your nails stronger? What about your hair? Some people notice new hair growth around this time. Also pay attention to your energy level. Are you still detoxing hard and needing more rest, or are you starting to feel stronger and more energized? These are all messages from your body. Keep listening. If you are not feeling any change at all, consult the Mid-Elimin8 Track Checkpoint on page 161 and follow the guidelines there for what to do next.

Indulge Yourself: Sleep More

Let's talk about sleep. Sleep is not a luxury. It is a mandate for your wellness. Sleep is essential for health. You heal and rejuvenate both body and mind when you sleep, yet many of us tend to make sleep a low priority. This week I want you to change that. Every day this week that you get even five minutes less than eight hours of sleep (which for most people is every day), I want you to do *either* of the following, depending on which fits into your schedule more (you might do each of them on different days):

- Brazenly take a 30-minute nap in the middle of the day. Turn off your phone, hang a DO NOT DISTURB sign on your door if necessary, get cozy, and snooze. Don't sleep longer than 30 minutes, so you aren't too groggy to keep going. You also don't want to make it harder to go to sleep at night.

- Go to bed one hour earlier than usual. Even if the kitchen isn't clean. Even if your show is still on (record it). Don't use that extra hour to look at your phone or watch TV. Dim the lights, maybe read a book, listen to music, or meditate for no more than 15 minutes, then snuggle in and get right down to the sleeping part. This might be easy for you. If your body genuinely needs more sleep, you might doze off in minutes. For others, sleep feels elusive. During your nap or earlier bedtime, you may feel wide awake because you aren't used to sleeping at that time. Persist. Your body will adjust because it craves sleep. You have to call its attention to the fact that sleep is what you are doing now. It's a habit like anything else (or, to be more accurate, resisting sleep is a habit). Deep breathing and counting your breaths can help. *No electronics!* The meditation or prayer you have been doing has also helped you train your mind to be calm. If you are still having trouble, here are some things to do to help yourself along:

- Holy basil (tulsi) is an adaptogenic herb that is excellent for calming the mind.

- Magnesium glycinate can also help to induce calm and sleep. Take magnesium before bed, according to package directions.

Sweet dreams!

Inflammatory Habit 4: Negativity

Did you know that you have around 60,000 thoughts every day? And what's even more surprising: One Stanford study found that a staggering 90 percent of those thoughts are repetitive.[17] Think about that: Nine out of ten of your thoughts are ones you have over and over again. For many people, these thoughts are not only repetitive but largely negative. Negative thoughts include things you are worried about, critical thoughts about your own appearance or abilities, dread of the future, regret about the past, etc. Negative thoughts fuel stress, and that is damaging to your overall health. I have seen people do their eliminations perfectly, but their improvement is stunted by constant negative thought patterns.

There may or may not be an "optimism gene,"[18] but whether you have it or feel like you broke yours years ago, it really is possible to train yourself out of the habit of negativity. I'm not suggesting you become a rose-colored-glasses type who blindly labels everything as "awesome." I am all for realism, but that is not the same as unrelenting negativity, which we know for sure has a not-so-hot effect on your health.[19] Negativity is inflammatory. It's not easy to change

Negativity is inflammatory.

your habitual way of relating to your own world, of course, but negativity is a habit, like anything else, so try giving it up today.

WHY GIVE IT UP (FOR NOW): Negativity is stressful. Anxiety, fear, worry, regret, pessimism, anger, and hate are some of the most common emotions that can keep you from reaching your health goals. Negative thoughts and emotions result in the release of stress hormones like cortisol, which have a measurable negative effect on your immune system.[20] Research consistently shows that people who have a more positive response to the events in their lives live longer, get sick less, recover more quickly, and are less likely to be depressed. They have healthier hearts and better coping skills.[21] Who wouldn't want some of that good medicine?

HOW TO GIVE IT UP: Mindful awareness will help you notice your negativity habit. Proceed slowly, consciously, and rationally. Be the observer of your own thoughts as if you're watching the thoughts of someone else scroll by. When do you tend to go negative? When is it easier to be positive? See if you can discern patterns and analyze the triggers to your negativity. Try to pinpoint what you might be holding on to from your past that's keeping you from your goals. Forgiving yourself and others can be a revolutionary act of healing. I consider this emotional healing to be vital in my work helping patients overcome their health obstacles. Negativity and positivity are habits, so today you are going to kick one to the curb and invite the other one into your life. Here are some tips.

WHAT TO DO INSTEAD: *No* is a habit. *Yes* is a habit. Work on catching yourself and then flipping what you were going to say to put a more positive spin on it. Consider it a personal challenge to your creativity.

ACTIVITIES TO INCORPORATE: Give these glass-half-full strategies a try.

- **Pay attention.** Start noticing your thoughts. When they are negative, question them. Ask yourself: *Is that true?*

- **Practice positivity.** Like any other skill, being more positive takes practice. Purposefully form positive thoughts, especially in response to negative thoughts. Even if you don't completely believe them, say them to yourself anyway. Fake it till you make it, as they say.

- **Notice your triggers.** If you are negative only in certain situations or with specific people, think about why. Can you change the situation? Is the relationship, environment, or situation something that can be fixed, or do you need to move on?

- **Laugh more.** Humor can be a good way to defuse negativity. Seek out chances to laugh more—funny friends, funny movies, or a willingness to be amused by the occasional absurdity of life.

- **Hang out with positive people.** When all your friends are Negative Nancys or Neds, it's easy to fall in step. When your friends tend to see the bright side, you are more likely to join in on that behavior.

- **Be patient with yourself.** Negativity is a hard habit to break, but be persistent. You may not conquer your negative habits *today*, but you can choose to make this the first day of the rest of your life when it comes to having a more positive outlook.

HOW DO YOU FEEL AFTER WEEK FOUR?

_____

_____

_____

_____

If you're on the Core4 track, you've reached a milestone. Proceed to chapter 7—and congratulate yourself on a job well done.

MID-ELIMIN8 TRACK CHECKPOINT

For the folks who are on the Elimin8 track—hurrah, you're halfway there! Although it has likely had its challenging moments, I bet you are feeling a lot different now—lighter, with more energy and reduced symptoms. However, a few of my patients at this point are still not experiencing symptom relief, even though they have been closely following the program. Not sure? This is the time to pull out that list of your top eight most bothersome symptoms, from page 54. Do you still have some of those? Are they still impeding your life? If that is you, then it is possible that you need a stronger intervention. At this point, you have two choices:

1. **Stay the course.** Some people with more inflammation, or whose systems are generally slower to react, may take longer to respond to the Elimin8 program, and patience may be warranted. Even though you may not be feeling it, your inflammation is reduced, if you have been following your plan. You may discover that by Week Five, Six, or Seven, you will suddenly enjoy a dramatic relief from your symptoms and start to feel better. Also, have you been cheating? If so, I encourage you to start over. Otherwise, stay the course and reassess after the eight weeks are over. I have more guidance for you then if you are still experiencing symptoms. Remember, bio-individuality means you won't react exactly like anyone else.

2. **Be more vigilant.** If you have been letting some things slip—a cheat here, a few extra portions there, a little of this or that that you think "couldn't really hurt"—it's time to tighten the reins. Give yourself the gift of 100 percent compliance for the next four weeks. It will make a big difference in accuracy when you begin to test the foods you

have eliminated. Remind yourself that you are forging a stronger and clearer communication with your body. Let's get this done. Elimin8 for the win!

ELIMIN8 WEEK FIVE

■ Before you begin, do your pre-week prep steps (page 126).

Your Typical Day

- This week, keep up with your increased morning meditation/ prayer/quiet time, and don't be tempted to skip mornings now. Even if you feel like you are noticing a difference already, research suggests that it takes four to six weeks to fully reap the benefits, so if you have been meditating consistently since Week One, you are almost due for noticing a change, like better sleep, less pain, improved circulation, better focus and problem solving, a better memory, and increased motivation, not to mention more empathy, calmness, better relationships, and a profound sense of well-being. The effects of meditation are cumulative, and over the course of a lifetime its benefits are profound.

- Eat your planned breakfast and pack up your lunch and a snack.

- Let's step it up another notch. Add one more tool from your toolbox. If you were already doing two of each, do three. If you were already doing three, try four. Not only is this another way to make your Elimin8 diet experience more effective, but the added foods and tools will also help keep things interesting. Even if you aren't sure you will like a new food or tool, it can't hurt to try. You don't have to keep doing it if it's not for you.

- Eat your planned lunch, snack, and dinner. Now that you are half done, you may be feeling the need to change up your meals. If you have gotten into the habit of a few favorite meals, shake it up this week. Try yet another recipe or invent a new meal or revamp an old favorite, using only foods from the allowed list at the beginning of this chapter. Keep planning ahead and have easy-to-prepare options so you won't be tempted by eliminated foods that will derail your significant progress.

- If weather permits, try exercising outside this week, if you normally don't. Or exercise somewhere else. Change the scenery or change up your routine. Try a different cardio machine. Try jogging if you've been walking. Check out the free weights if you use weight machines or start lifting some light weights if you haven't been doing that. If you like sports, you could also look into a local team or class. How about tennis or pickleball lessons? A racquetball league? A running club? Or maybe yoga, Pilates, or a dance class is more your speed. After four weeks, your body should be ready for an increased physical challenge, and you probably have more fitness confidence, so this is a good time to take it to the next level.

- Do one replacement behavior each day for your inflammatory habit of the week.

- Before bed, meditate for as long as you did in the morning. Remember your mantra, which may be running in your head all the time by now, but also be open to new techniques. What about visualization? When you meditate, create a place in your mind of ultimate calm. It might be a place you've been or a place you imagine—a beach, a forest, a Zen grotto, a riverbank, a luxury retreat for one somewhere far away. Let it be a place or vision that inspires you. Imagine yourself there and try to visualize all the details of what you see, hear, smell, and feel. There is no limit to where you can imagine yourself.

WEEK FIVE MEAL PLAN

	BREAKFAST	ELIXIR
MONDAY		
TUESDAY		
WEDNESDAY		
THURSDAY		
FRIDAY		
SATURDAY		
SUNDAY		

LUNCH	SNACK	DINNER

Your Weekly Pep Talk

I hope you are feeling pretty good about your Elimin8 stamina so far. You've been doing things that you might not have believed you could do, and you've been doing them for a whole month. You rock. This week let's continue strong and get social. According to research,[22] spending time with friends and having an active social life could extend your life, improve your physical and mental health, and even lower your risk of dementia as you age. Organize that girls' or guys' night out (have fun with your virgin cocktails, yes?), meet a friend for tea, or take more time to hang with family members and catch up on how things are going for them. People tend to get so wrapped up in their busy schedules that they forget to check in with their partners, kids, siblings, or parents. We all need to share with other people. We are social animals. Let yourself be there for someone and let someone be there for you. The more you engage directly with the external world, the better you will feel, I promise.

And what if you feel like you don't have anyone to do this with? Some people live far from family or are estranged. Others have recently relocated and don't know anyone yet or may be so busy with work that they haven't had time to cultivate a social network. If that is you, then make this your week to reach out. Skype or FaceTime faraway friends and relatives, or look around for local opportunities to meet people, like places of worship, social meet-up groups of people who share a common interest (find these online), or local gatherings like festivals, concerts, farmers markets, or community classes. Be open to making new friends. You might not meet anyone in particular, but an open friendliness will make the experience more fun, and you never know what could happen. This is the kind of daring leap that can make you feel braver and stronger, and it also fulfills a biological need to exist within a community. Get out there and let people meet your lovable self.

Indulge Yourself: Friend Time

This week play hooky on a weekday. (Ask permission first. I don't want you to lose your job.) Meet a good friend, a family member, or someone you want to get to know better for a late-morning or midafternoon cup of hot tea and a friendly chat. You could also take an extended lunch hour to do this, or if that's impossible, make time on the weekend. Relax and just be with someone else for an hour.

Inflammatory Habit 5: Monkey Mind

Monkey mind comes from a Buddhist term (both Chinese and Japanese have versions of it) meaning "unsettled" or "capricious," and it is used to mean a restless mind that can't concentrate because it keeps jumping around like a crazy monkey, unable to settle on any subject or engage in any deep thought. This anxious, reactive mind is prevalent in our culture, which is so often focused on sound bites, video clips, advertisements, and other visual and aural stimuli that change constantly to draw and keep our attention.

WHY GIVE IT UP (FOR NOW): The result of chronic monkey mind is that we have trouble paying attention to anything for longer than about 30 seconds (or less!). Monkey mind also describes that state when you lie awake in bed at night thinking of a million things you need to do or worrying about a long list of things that probably won't ever happen. How can you possibly have a restful sleep with all that ruckus going on?

HOW TO GIVE IT UP: A crucial step to resolving, or at least significantly taming, your monkey mind is to become aware that we spend much of our day lost in compulsive thought. Remember that for most of us, nine out of ten of our thoughts are ones we have repeatedly, so really, what a waste of time! You won't get rid of that monkey in your brain in one day, but today is a chance to begin taming it with awareness. That monkey doesn't want you to notice him, but once you do, you've got the upper hand.

WHAT TO DO INSTEAD: Detachment from the reactive thinking mind is liberating and calming to your system. You are not your thoughts or your emotions, but the observing presence of them. As you go through the day, become aware of when your mind starts jumping around. Noticing is the first step. When you notice, see if you can detach from the "jumping around" so that you feel like you are looking at it from the outside rather than being in the thick of it. This might feel hard at first, but with practice, you will get better and better. The trick is consistency. Once you get the hang of this, you will likely find that it is relaxing to step outside your chaotic thoughts and calmly observe them without getting roped back into your own mental drama.

ACTIVITIES TO INCORPORATE: This exercise will help train your mental monkeys into submission:

- Two times today, for at least 5 minutes each (ideally once first thing in the morning and once right before going to bed), sit quietly without disturbances and focus on thinking about one thing. It can be an image, a word, a sound, or a concept like love or peace.

- When your mind jumps around like a little rascally monkey, patiently bring it back to your one thing. (It's not unlike training a puppy.) Breathe slowly and deeply while you do this and let your mind rest.

- Do this every day, and when you master 5 minutes, increase your sessions by a minute. When you've mastered 6 minutes, increase the time again until you are calmly thinking of one thing for 15 minutes twice a day. Monkey mind: mastered.

———

HOW DO YOU FEEL AFTER WEEK FIVE? Are your symptoms continuing to decrease? Are some totally gone? Stay the course! You can't always feel all the inflammation in your system, so keep going to continue dousing those flames. Summarize your current mental and physical health state:

_____

_____

_____

_____

_____

ELIMIN8 WEEK SIX

■ Before you begin, do your pre-week prep steps (page 126).

Your Typical Day

- This week increase your morning meditation, prayer, or quiet time by yet another 5 minutes. If you started at 5 minutes, you should be up to 15 minutes by now. If you started at 10 minutes, you should be up to 20, and so forth. I won't ask you to bump it up any more than this, but keep increasing the time if you like. Some people meditate for an hour or even more each day. However, 15 to 20 minutes each morning and evening makes for an excellent practice that will give you a lifetime of benefits.

- Enjoy your planned breakfast and pack up your lunch and snack. You are ready for any eating challenge that comes your way today.

WEEK SIX MEAL PLAN

	BREAKFAST	ELIXIR
MONDAY		
TUESDAY		
WEDNESDAY		
THURSDAY		
FRIDAY		
SATURDAY		
SUNDAY		

LUNCH	SNACK	DINNER

- Keep up with your three tools from your toolbox. These will continue to reduce inflammation. Is your body still talking to you? Is it telling you how it's doing? At this point, if you react positively or negatively to some food you try or something you do, you will probably be much better able to hear the message. If you hear it, heed it.

- Eat your planned lunch, snack, and dinner. Is your new way of eating beginning to feel like a healthy habit?

- Keep up with your exercise this week. It should be feeling like something you do now, and that's great. Have you noticed a difference in body shape, strength, mood, and energy? (Don't weigh yourself yet!) Pay attention to how your body responds during and after exercise. It's talking to you. Let it tell you what it likes and doesn't like about your movement choices.

- Keep up with your inflammatory habit replacement behavior of the week.

- Before bed, increase your meditation, prayer, or quiet time by 5 minutes. Can you match the time you spent in the morning? If you fall asleep while trying to meditate in the evening, that is fine. It means your body was calm enough to sleep and needed to sleep, and since you are listening so well now, you know that you should let it sleep.

Your Weekly Pep Talk

Wow, how did you get to Week Six already? Or maybe it seems like it's been forever. In either case, this week I want you to think about staying the course. Your new habits are getting more and more established as your old habits are fading further from your consciousness. Habits can be like ruts in the road, places where your wheel always tends to go. It's hard to pop your wheel out of that rut and start driving on the flat part of the road, but once you're out of that rut, the driving will be easier. When your good habits become established, it will be harder to quit them than it will be to go back to the bad ones. Keep steering clear of those old ways. Good riddance. Stay strong this week with everything you are doing for yourself—body, mind, and soul.

Indulge Yourself: Eat Out

This week, I want you to take a leap and go out to eat. Maybe you've avoided this so far because you aren't sure what you will be getting when you order, and you don't want to annoy the server. Maybe your job requires that you go out to eat often but not necessarily for pleasure. In either case, this week, choose a nice place with high-quality food and a dining companion (or several) that you love to be around. Find the menu online (or visit the restaurant ahead of time) and find some options that look good to you, made up mostly of your *yes* foods. Then arrange with the restaurant (ahead of time if your request is complex) to make your meal 100 percent Elimin8 compliant. You don't need to overexplain. For best results, just call ahead and tell the restaurant you are on a special diet for health reasons. Most chefs at good restaurants, especially those with a natural-food or locavore bent, are more than happy to work with you to create a delicious dish you can enjoy without worry. Give it a try. If you are timid, maybe a friend can help with the call or the in-person request.

When you are at the restaurant, tell your server that you have made arrangements for a meal and be specific about what you need, even if you have already spoken to a manager or the chef previously. Don't assume there is complete communication between chefs and servers when the restaurant gets busy. Then sit back, enjoy your food fully, relish your dining companions, soak in the restaurant's atmosphere, and let the whole experience wash over you. Your meal is on plan, so all you have to do is relax and enjoy. Most of all, have a great time. Pleasure is anti-inflammatory.

Inflammatory Habit 6: Emotional Eating

Emotional eating, sometimes called stress eating, is a stress response that involves consuming food to relieve stress, distract yourself from unpleasant feelings, or provide a little moment of pleasure in the face of depression or anxiety. In other words, when you feel bad, you eat to feel better. It's the proverbial pint-of-ice-cream-after-a-breakup scenario. Eating for reasons other than hunger is okay now and then—to celebrate, to socialize. However, if eating for emotional reasons becomes chronic—you do it more than a few times a week, or even daily—then it is a problem and can damage your health. It isn't about eating for hunger. It is about eating your feelings, and that's not a healthy physical or emotional practice.

When you have emotional "hunger," food will not fill you. It is only a temporary distraction that will likely leave you feeling even worse later, especially if it causes you to go against the health improvements you've been trying so hard to make. The kinds of foods emotional eaters usually crave are high in refined carbs like sugar and white flour or fried like potato chips or French fries or extremely high in fat like cheese, or all of the above, like a doughnut. One intense emotional eating session can derail your good health efforts, so if you are an emotional eater and want to feel better, you will benefit immensely by working through this problem.

WHY GIVE IT UP (FOR NOW): Emotional eating can cause uncomfortable weight gain and digestive problems like bloating and reflux. It can lead to an eating disorder like compulsive overeating or bulimia (some people believe emotional eating itself *is* an eating disorder). It can trigger blood sugar irregularities, cause nutritional deficiencies, and make anxiety and depression worse, not better.

HOW TO GIVE IT UP: If you are an emotional eater, you probably already know you aren't going to solve this problem in one day, but you *can* solve it by gradually increasing your awareness of the cues that make you feel like eating. Emotional eating has complex roots and can be tough to overcome, but today you can begin by making a rule for yourself: Don't eat anything when you are upset or anxious. Always wait to eat until you feel calm. (That monkey mind exercise can help you now.) If you eat when you are having a negative emotion, you are likely to have problems properly and fully digesting your food because of the gut-brain axis: Your gut knows what your brain is thinking, and negative emotions are stressful. Stress means the body directs its resources away from the gut to other parts of the body to handle the stress. To help you break the habit of eating when your body isn't prepared for food, try these two steps:

1. Resolve to eat only when you feel calm. This can make a big difference in breaking the habit of reaching for a cookie or a bag of chips with every emotional downturn.

2. Once you are calm and feel ready to eat, before putting even one bite of food in your mouth, take one deep, long, slow breath, focus on the food, and then eat it slowly. Notice everything about the experience. Don't look at your phone, don't read anything, don't watch television. The next time you eat, do this again. And do it once more every time you eat anything at all, even a snack, even one nibble. This will help you catch yourself when you are starting to eat emotionally, as emotional eating often happens mindlessly.

The point of this exercise is to help you make food about food, and about nothing but food. You can't get rid of strong emotions, and this isn't about repressing your feelings or judging your emotions. Emotions come and go. This practice is about disassociating feelings about other things in your life from the food you eat, thus processing your emotions separately from processing your food.

Do the above two things from now on, every day and every time you eat. Sometimes you might forget or eat without doing this when your emotions hijack your good intentions, but when you do, be patient with yourself. Gently remind yourself to come back to this exercise, with love and compassion for yourself and for the strong feelings you are having.

WHAT TO DO INSTEAD: Negative emotions, especially anxiety, can make you feel compelled to *do something, anything,* to relieve the bad feeling. Food is an easy response, but there are many other things you can do, and if you don't find something else to replace your automatic eating response, it will be harder to overcome it. Make a list of five things you like to do that you can do immediately without any preparation, and post the list in your kitchen or wherever you are most likely to see it when you have the urge to eat emotionally. Pick one of those things and decide, firmly, to do that instead.

ACTIVITIES TO INCORPORATE: Here are activities to substitute for emotional eating. Your list will of course reflect your own preferences.

- Listen to three favorite songs in a row with headphones.

- Go for a walk—no need to change clothes, just go.

- Take 20 slow deep breaths, counting to 5 as you inhale and 10 as you exhale.

- Take a shower and vigorously scrub all your skin with a brush or washcloth, then moisturize everywhere.

- Sit down and watch a funny show or movie (no food or cell phone—just be present for the show).

- Drink 16 ounces of water.

- Eat four stalks of celery—although it's food, it's not a "binge" food, and the crunch can help relieve anxiety.

- Take a 20-minute catnap.

- Free-write for 15 minutes without stopping. Write whatever you are feeling without thinking about it or worrying about grammar or how it sounds. No judgment—it's just for you.

- Do anything else that relieves the pressure of your immediate in-the-moment feeling that *doesn't* involve food.

When to Seek Help

For some people, eating issues require a professional, and there is nothing wrong with that. A therapist trained in eating issues can help you to identify the source of your emotional eating and give you strategies for extricating your emotions from your eating behavior and finding more effective and personalized ways to handle your emotions.

HOW DO YOU FEEL AFTER WEEK SIX? You have only two more weeks to go. What physical and mental health improvements have you noticed this week?

_____

_____

_____

_____

ELIMIN8 WEEK SEVEN

■ Before you begin, do your pre-week prep steps (page 126).

Your Typical Day

- Homestretch alert! You have only two weeks left. Can you believe it? Now is the time to start thinking about how you want to incorporate these morning meditation/prayer/quiet time sessions into the rest of your life. Are you feeling benefits? Do you love it yet? Does your body tell you that it loves this ritual? If so, think about how to do this every morning from now on. And if you are still on the fence? If you aren't sure your body cares that much? Keep going with it. Don't skip a day. By the end of the eight weeks, I hope you will be convinced, but if not, then proceed according to your natural inclinations.

- You have just two weeks left, so this is a good time to start thinking about how you can carry this meal-planning habit with you into the rest of your life. You know what the scouts say: Be prepared.

- Let's up the ante one more time. For the next two weeks, try to include at least *four* tools from your toolbox, or one more than you have already been doing, to squash any remaining stubborn inflammation with the big guns.

- Keep going with your exercise. Keep changing it up, if that makes things more interesting. Make a long-term commitment, such as signing up for a league or an extended class or session at a gym, studio, or with a group. This will help keep your habit going, even after your elimination journey is over. Also stay in tune with what your body loves and hates about exercise. Everyone is different and responds differently. Some people need more vigorous activity and some people need more calming activity, while most people probably do best with a combination of both. Can you tell which your body prefers?

- If you still have inflammatory habits you want to boot out of your life, do the replacement behaviors for the one you choose to eliminate this week.

- Again, keep up with your evening ritual and think about how you can keep this up after this program ends, or if you want to keep it up. Do you notice sleep and/or brain benefits? Think about what you want to do going forward. (Don't think for too long—you've got sleeping to do.)

Your Weekly Pep Talk

What, only one more week after this one? Time sure flies when you're living that anti-inflammatory life. I'm so proud of you and everything you've accomplished up to this point. This week, I want you to start thinking about what to do after this program is over. Which habits, practices, foods, recipes, and attitudes do you want to keep forever? Which do you want to keep in your back pocket in case you need to pull them out and use them as needed? Which aren't working for you? Get your mind oriented toward the future, but don't let that distract you from staying strong on the plan right now. You've got this week and next week to go, and then you get to start testing by reintegrating the foods you've given up. You may end up bringing some old favorites back in, but that doesn't mean you should abandon the rest of this anti-inflammatory lifestyle. Keep listening to your body, because it will help you make all of these decisions.

WEEK SEVEN MEAL PLAN

	BREAKFAST	ELIXIR
MONDAY		
TUESDAY		
WEDNESDAY		
THURSDAY		
FRIDAY		
SATURDAY		
SUNDAY		

LUNCH	SNACK	DINNER

Indulge Yourself: Spa Day, Optionally DIY

This week you deserve a spa day. Pick one day, and line up some spa services, such as a massage, a mani-pedi, a wash and blowout (or getting your gray hairs colored, if that's your thing), a wax, a Reiki session, an infrared sauna, a soak in a Jacuzzi, or whatever you most enjoy. This can be as simple or as elaborate as you want to make it. If you can't or don't want to go to an actual spa, you could do a DIY spa day on your own. Relax in a warm bath full of Epsom salts and essential oils (lavender, rose, and ylang-ylang are good oil choices for relaxation), with candles and music. Trade massages with a partner or friend. Soak and scrub your feet and do your nails, if you enjoy that. Wash your hair and do that thing you do to it that takes a long time but is worth it. Go to a local pool with a hot tub and soak there. Or take an hour to relax, put your feet up, listen to music you love, and chill out. Let it feel luxurious. You've earned it.

Inflammatory Habit 7: Social Isolation and/or Social Media Addiction

Humans are social beings, no doubt, but relationships and human communication can be difficult, even painful. What better remedy than removing the human from the equation? Social media can be a fun way to keep in touch with old friends or share the daily details of your life with people from your past or those who live far away, but when it becomes your primary social activity, you may have a problem. Social media engineers have created those programs to be addictive. They take advantage of FOMO (that's "fear of missing out," folks). What if you miss something big happening in the world? What if you miss what happened to someone? What if *people miss you?* When someone likes something you posted or comments positively, it releases dopamine,[23] like a drug. It makes you feel so good. *They like me. They really like me.*

WHY GIVE IT UP (FOR NOW): Social media keeps people constantly interrupted as they continually stop what they are doing to check their notifications. This keeps them from ever being fully engaged in an activity for an extended period—a skill you can lose if you never practice it. Social media also makes human communication less empathetic. People say things on social media they probably wouldn't say in person. This can result in bullying, hate speech, oversimplification of complex issues, divisiveness, and ultimately, depression and isolation from actual human contact.[24] Social media can also strain your actual relationships with friends and family—even make your partner and kids feel like you care more about your phone than you care about them. Is that really what you want to do?

HOW TO GIVE IT UP: There are several popular trends out there to help people quit, or at least take a break, challenging people to go an amount of time—ninety-nine days, a month, even one day—without social media. At first people who try this report feeling lost, but soon they begin to regain their lives and lost social skills. Are you game to try it?

Today—for *today only*—stay off social media completely. Work emails are fine, but no Facebook, no Twitter, no Instagram, no Snapchat, no Pinterest, no Reddit, no LinkedIn, no Myspace (just kidding), no Tumblr, no Google, and no, not even Tinder. No swiping left *or* right today. Transform your FOMO into JOMO ("joy of missing out"). Consider it a psychology experiment on yourself. You may be amazed at how much you are able to wake up to the physical world around you in just one day. You can check back in tomorrow, but I hope you'll keep doing this periodically—such as one social-media-free day per week—even after your Elimin8 time is over.

WHAT TO DO INSTEAD: Many people have literal withdrawal symptoms from not being able to hold and check their phones— yeah, this is a problem. It helps to have a replacement behavior. When you feel nervous or lost or compelled to check your social media, that is a sign from your brain that you need actual human connection. Reward your brain with a more fulfilling activity.

ACTIVITIES TO INCORPORATE: Try these strategies to help you reconnect with actual face-to-face humans again.

- Have a conversation with a friend or family member who is physically with you.

- Better yet, spend the day with a real person, in a no-phone zone, talking about your lives.

- Write a letter using a pen and some paper. Mail it in a real envelope with an actual stamp. So retro!

- Notice whether your other family members have a problem, too—you could make this "social media cleanse" a family affair or challenge, especially since many kids and teens have problems with this issue.

HOW DO YOU FEEL AFTER WEEK SEVEN? One more week to go! Do you feel like you have met some or all of your goals?

_____

_____

_____

_____

ELIMIN8 WEEK EIGHT

■ Before you begin, do your pre-week prep steps (page 126).

Your Typical Day

- Incredibly, you are in your last week, but this is no time to slack off. You are not done until the last day of your eighth week, so stick with everything you've been doing, and do it with extra fervor—let's finish strong. That means meditating, praying, or sitting quietly every single morning this week. Also look back on how far you've come and look forward to all the amazing things you have ahead of you. Meditate on that! And remember that good old mantra? Say it with gusto this week.

- This is your last week of structured meal planning. Starting next week, you will begin reintroducing some foods you haven't had in a long while. To get the best answer from your body next week when you do that, it is important that no inflammation sneaks back in this week, so stay 100 percent true to your food list.

- This is your last week of prescribed tools from your toolbox, but use these any time you feel you need them. These targeted resources are always available as your secret weapons if your symptoms of inflammation ever creep back in.

- Keep moving this week. Exercise is a part of your natural life now.

- If you have one more inflammatory habit you want to break, go hard this week. If any one of the other seven inflammatory habits has crept back in, look back and reinstitute those replacement behaviors. Ingrained habits are hard to break and take time, so I don't expect you to be perfectly over all of these, but continued vigilance and listening to your body will help you keep cultivating better habits.

- Before bed each night, let your meditation, prayers, or thoughts focus on gratitude. Who has helped you in your elimination

WEEK EIGHT MEAL PLAN

	BREAKFAST	ELIXIR
MONDAY		
TUESDAY		
WEDNESDAY		
THURSDAY		
FRIDAY		
SATURDAY		
SUNDAY		

LUNCH	SNACK	DINNER

journey? A family member? A friend? A doctor or health-care practitioner? A support group or therapist? New people you met during the last eight weeks? What do you have in your life that has allowed you to do this program—a supportive partner or cheerleader friend? Financial resources? A flexible job? Gratitude is anti-inflammatory, and it also helps us keep our own lives in perspective. Life and health are journeys, and we don't go through them alone.

Your Weekly Pep Talk

Cue the trumpets. Bang the drums. You are in your last week. This is the time to pat yourself on the back and sail through without a hitch. This week, stay strong with everything you are doing. No quitting early. I would also like you to look back to what you wrote during the eight days you were stepping down through your eliminated items, and also what you wrote after the first week. Think back to that time. What has changed? Sometimes when changes are gradual, we don't notice them until we remember how we used to feel. How did you feel before you started this program?

Every single thing that has changed during the last eight weeks is a communication from your body. This is important to understand. If you feel better and certain symptoms are reduced or gone, your body is telling you that it loves something (or everything) that you have been doing—or not doing. If certain symptoms are still hanging around, that is also a message from your body, either that it still dislikes something you are doing or that it isn't done healing yet. All of this is good information, so this week, listen, listen, listen. You need to be closely tuned in before reintegrating eliminated foods, so put the finishing touches on your body listening skills. You're about to use them intensively. (And still no weighing yourself—you can do that next week, or if you don't care, skip it altogether.)

Indulge Yourself: Give Yourself a Gift

This week, give yourself a gift to reward yourself for all your hard work. It can be a new piece of clothing (possibly in a smaller size), an accessory like a scarf, tie, jewelry, or a new wallet, or something else you've been wanting, like stationery, a cool crystal, a candle, or a gadget. It can also be an experience, a service, or simply a day off. It can be big or small, expensive or completely free. It can be new or used, but it should be something you wouldn't normally indulge in. Imagine that you're picking out something your best friend would truly love and cherish, filled with all the love you have for her or him. Maybe wrap it. Maybe even add a card, where you write to your friend (you) about everything she or he means to you. Make it a little over the top. You've earned it.

Inflammatory Habit 8: Lack of Higher Purpose

This last inflammatory habit is a little more philosophical. Today I would like you to consider what your higher purpose is in this life. You may know immediately, and that's great. Or you may need to think about it for a while. You may even realize you don't have one yet. If you don't have one, it's time to start figuring this out, because once you understand the benefits of living and thriving in the service of something greater than yourself, you will be motivated to continue your health journey.

What do I mean by higher purpose? It could be a spiritual practice. It could be a mission in life. It could be something you love to do more than anything else, something that gets you up in the morning. Whatever it may be, it's what gives your life meaning.

WHY HAVE A HIGHER PURPOSE? Having a higher purpose has been demonstrated to improve health, recovery from illness or surgery, and brain function, including stroke risk.[25] It is deeply connected to your well-being. Those who report not having a higher purpose tend to have poorer outcomes after a health crisis, more depression, and less life satisfaction.

HOW DO YOU GET ONE? I would like you to think hard about this during this last week. What gives your life meaning? Do you actively believe in something bigger than yourself? If your life had a mission statement, what would it include? If you already know some answers, put them in the forefront of your mind. Try writing a mission statement. It doesn't have to be long, but it can help you clarify your priorities. What is your life about? If you aren't sure, just keep the question in your mind. Keep asking yourself the question. Something will eventually emerge, and it may change over time, but whatever it is right now, that is something to prioritize.

ACTIVITIES TO INCORPORATE: Here are some things to do to help you discover your higher purpose—they are long-term things, but take just one step toward making at least one of these happen this week:

- Join a place of worship or a spiritual group or study some spiritual tradition that interests you.

- Learn something new that you have always wanted to learn, such as how to play the piano, or how to speak Spanish, French, Italian, Chinese, or how to do karate or tai chi or yoga, or how to knit or do woodworking. It doesn't have to be lofty (although it could be). It just has to get you feeling passionate. You can try multiple activities to see what resonates with you.

- Pick up something you used to love but stopped doing when life got in the way. Maybe you could start planning that trip you've been wanting to take, or finish that book you started writing, or finally get that degree. If you used to dance or write poetry or paint landscapes or play the guitar and you loved it, carve out a time to start doing it again.

- You could volunteer with an organization that helps others—children, animals, the hungry, the poor, whatever it is that catches your heart—and see how service work changes your perspective.

When you find it, you will know it. Tell yourself about it here:

_____

_____

_____

_____

HOW DO YOU FEEL AFTER WEEK EIGHT? You've *done* it, and now you have the chance to look back over the last eight weeks and consider your progress. What has changed about your life? Now that you have completed your Elimin8 phase, move on to chapter 7 to learn how to reintegrate the foods we took a break from for eight weeks.

_____

_____

_____

_____

6

DEDIC8: YOUR ANTI-INFLAMMATORY COOKBOOK

No matter what foods you are putting on hold for the next four or eight weeks, enjoy all the things you get to eat with these safe and deeply nourishing recipes. In this mini cookbook, you will find Core4 track recipes, then Elimin8 track recipes. After these, look for the section on superfood elixirs as well as broths, which some of the recipes in this book use but which can also be sipped on their own.

The meal plans starting on page 122 use all these recipes, but you can pick and choose according to your tastes, trying out the ones that look good to you and ignoring those that don't. Or be adventurous and try them all! If you don't normally have time to cook during the week, most of these recipes can be made ahead and stored in the refrigerator or freezer for quick weekday meals. Everything is here to help you, not limit you. You can always adapt any of these recipes to suit you, or pick and choose the ones that look good and ignore the others.

NOTE: Whenever a recipe ingredient says "compliant," that means it is a food that has been premade (such as chicken apple sausage or mayonnaise) and all ingredients in it must be compliant with your food list, with no ingredients on your list of eliminated foods. If you buy any packaged foods, read the labels carefully.

CORE4 RECIPES
Core4 Breakfasts

....

Coconut–Butternut Squash Porridge

Start to finish: 10 minutes

Serves 2 to 3

1 (10-ounce) package frozen cubed butternut squash

¼ cup canned unsweetened coconut milk, plus additional milk for serving

½ teaspoon ground cinnamon

¼ teaspoon grated orange peel

⅓ cup pomegranate seeds

¼ cup chopped walnuts, toasted

1. Cook the butternut squash in a microwave oven according to the package directions. Transfer the squash to a medium bowl. Mash with a potato masher until smooth. Stir in the ¼ cup coconut milk, cinnamon, and orange peel.

2. Cover the bowl with a paper towel; microwave on high for 2 minutes or until heated through, stirring once halfway through heating.

3. Spoon the porridge into bowls. If desired, drizzle with additional coconut milk. Top with the pomegranate seeds and walnuts.

Fluffy Grain-Free Pancakes

Start to finish: 20 minutes

Serves 4

½ cup cassava flour

½ cup coconut flour

1 teaspoon ground cinnamon

⅛ teaspoon kosher salt

1 teaspoon aluminum-free baking powder

1 teaspoon orange zest or lemon zest (optional)

¾ to 1 cup almond milk, hemp milk, or coconut milk

1 ripe banana, mashed

2 large eggs

1 teaspoon vanilla extract

1 tablespoon coconut oil, plus additional as needed

Toppings, such as ghee, blueberries, sliced strawberries, sliced bananas, and/or whipped unsweetened coconut cream* (optional)

1. In a medium bowl, whisk together the cassava and coconut flours, cinnamon, salt, baking powder, and orange zest, if using; set aside.

2. In a blender container, combine the almond milk, banana, eggs, and vanilla. Cover and blend until smooth. Pour the almond milk mixture into the flour mixture. Whisk until smooth.

3. In a cast-iron griddle or heavy large skillet, heat the 1 tablespoon coconut oil over medium heat. Pour about ¼ cup batter at a time onto the griddle, spreading the batter if necessary. Cook for 2 minutes or until bubbles form on top and bottom is golden brown. Turn the pancakes and cook for 1 to 2 minutes more or until the bottom is golden. (Add more coconut oil to the pan as needed.)

4. Serve warm with toppings, if desired.

*NOTE: This is a canned product and is thicker than coconut milk. Use only unsweetened varieties. The cream that rises to the top of a can of full-fat coconut milk is also coconut cream. If you can't find unsweetened coconut cream, you can use that.

Hummus and Greens Breakfast Bowl

Start to finish: 30 minutes

Serves 4

3 tablespoons olive oil or avocado oil

1 tablespoon white wine vinegar

1 teaspoon compliant Dijon mustard

1 tablespoon finely chopped
shallot

⅛ teaspoon kosher salt

Coarse freshly ground black
pepper

1 (5-ounce) container power
greens or other mixed
greens

Zucchini Hummus (page 218)

2 cups leftover shredded chicken
or pork, or ¼ cup crumbled
cooked bacon, or 4 soft-
boiled eggs

1 to 2 tablespoons sunflower
seeds, toasted

Red pepper flakes (optional)

1. For the vinaigrette, in a small bowl, whisk together the oil,
   vinegar, mustard, shallot, salt, and pepper to taste. Place the greens
   in a large bowl; lightly drizzle with the vinaigrette and toss to coat.

2. Smear some of the hummus in each of four shallow bowls. Place the
   greens on top of the hummus. Top the greens with ½ cup chicken
   or pork, 1 tablespoon crumbled cooked bacon, or 1 egg. Sprinkle
   with sunflower seeds, and red pepper flakes, if using.

Mexican Avocado Baked Eggs

Start to finish: 25 minutes
Serves 4

2 large ripe avocados

4 large eggs

¼ teaspoon ground cumin

⅛ teaspoon kosher salt

1 cup chopped red and/or yellow
grape tomatoes

¼ cup finely chopped red
onion

1 tablespoon finely chopped fresh
cilantro

2 teaspoons fresh lime juice

1. Preheat the oven to 425°F. Cut the avocados lengthwise in half;
   remove the pits. Scoop out the flesh, leaving ½-inch-thick shells. Set
   aside the avocado flesh.

2. Place each avocado half in a muffin cup or ramekin. Crack one egg
   at a time into a custard cup or small bowl and pour only what fits

into the avocado; discard the leftover egg white. Sprinkle the eggs with ground cumin and salt. Bake for 15 to 20 minutes or until whites have set and the yolks begin to thicken.

3. Meanwhile, for the salsa, coarsely chop the avocado flesh. In a small bowl, combine the chopped avocado, tomatoes, onion, cilantro, and lime juice. Top the baked avocado eggs with the salsa.

Nuts, Seeds, and Coconut Granola

Prep: 15 minutes
Bake: 20–25 minutes
Serves 6 to 8

4 Medjool dates, pitted

3 tablespoons coconut oil

1 teaspoon vanilla extract

1 teaspoon ground cinnamon

½ teaspoon sea salt

1 cup almonds

1 cup pecans

1 cup walnuts

½ cup unsweetened coconut flakes

¼ cup sunflower seeds

¼ cup pumpkin seeds (pepitas)

1. Preheat the oven to 325°F. In a small bowl, combine the dates and enough hot water to cover. Let the dates soak for 10 minutes. Drain the dates; discard soaking water. Place the soaked dates and coconut oil in a food processor; process until a paste forms. Add the vanilla, cinnamon, and salt. Process until combined.

2. Add the almonds, pecans, and walnuts to the date mixture in the food processor. Pulse a few times to combine.

3. Line a large baking pan with foil. Spread the granola on the foil. Sprinkle the granola with the coconut flakes, sunflower seeds, and pumpkin seeds. Bake for 20 to 25 minutes or until toasted and beginning to crisp.

4. Remove the pan from the oven and let cool completely.

Spiced Mushroom and Veggie Hash with Sunshine Eggs

Prep: 20 minutes

Roast: 30 minutes

Serves 4

2 (8-ounce) packages sliced button mushrooms

2 medium carrots, peeled and chopped

12 small Yukon gold potatoes, quartered

1 cup chopped shallots

3 tablespoons olive oil

1 teaspoon ground cumin

½ teaspoon ground cinnamon

½ teaspoon smoked paprika

1 teaspoon kosher salt

½ teaspoon freshly ground black pepper

4 cups lightly packed baby kale, spinach, or arugula

4 large eggs*

Chopped fresh flat-leaf parsley (optional)

1. Preheat the oven to 450°F. Position a rack in the center of the oven. Line a large baking pan with parchment paper or foil.

2. In a large bowl, combine the mushrooms, carrots, potatoes, and shallots. In a small bowl, stir together the olive oil, cumin, cinnamon, paprika, salt, and pepper. Pour over the vegetables and stir to coat. Spread the vegetables on the baking pan. Roast for 20 minutes or until the potatoes are just tender and starting to brown.

3. Reduce the oven temperature to 400°F. Add the kale to the pan and stir until it wilts; return the pan to the oven for 2 to 3 minutes if necessary.

4. Make four indentations in the hash and carefully break one egg into each indentation. Roast the hash for 8 to 10 minutes more, or until the egg whites are set and the yolks are desired doneness. Top with the parsley, if using.

*NOTE: To make this dish vegan, omit the eggs.

Sweet Potato Breakfast Skillet

Prep: 15 minutes

Cook: 15 minutes

Serves 4

3 tablespoons ghee or olive oil, divided

1 pound sweet potatoes, peeled, quartered lengthwise, and sliced ¼ inch thick

1 cup sliced cremini mushrooms

1 small yellow onion, chopped

½ cup chopped red bell pepper

½ teaspoon kosher salt

½ teaspoon smoked paprika

¼ teaspoon freshly ground black pepper

2 fully cooked compliant chicken-and-apple sausage links (sugar free), quartered lengthwise and cut into ¼-inch slices

2 cups sliced kale

4 large eggs

1. In a 12-inch cast-iron skillet, heat 2 tablespoons of the ghee over medium heat until hot. Add the sweet potatoes in a single layer. Cover and cook for 6 to 8 minutes, turning the potatoes halfway through cooking.

2. Add the mushrooms, onion, bell pepper, salt, paprika, and pepper; gently toss to combine. Cook, uncovered, for 3 minutes. Add the sausage and kale; cook, uncovered, for 3 to 5 minutes or until the kale is wilted and the vegetables are tender.

3. Meanwhile, in a large nonstick skillet, heat the remaining 1 tablespoon ghee over medium heat. Break the eggs into the skillet. Reduce the heat to low; cook for 3 to 4 minutes or until the whites are set and the yolks begin to thicken.

4. Divide the sweet potato mixture among four plates. Top each serving with a fried egg.

Core4 Lunches
....

Garlicky Butternut Squash Noodles with Kielbasa

Start to finish: 20 minutes
Serves 2 to 3

2 tablespoons olive oil or ghee

2 garlic cloves, thinly sliced

1 (12-ounce) package fresh or frozen butternut squash noodles

2 compliant (sugar-free) kielbasa sausages or chicken-apple sausages, sliced

1 cup packed baby spinach, arugula, or kale

Kosher salt and freshly ground black pepper

¼ cup coarsely chopped toasted pecans

1. In a large skillet, heat olive oil over medium-high heat. Add the garlic; cook for 1 minute or until golden, stirring frequently. Transfer the garlic to small bowl; set aside. Add the butternut squash noodles to the hot skillet. Cook, covered, for 5 minutes, stirring occasionally. Add the kielbasa to the skillet. Cook, covered, for 5 minutes more or until the sausage is heated through and noodles are tender.

2. Return the garlic to the skillet. Gently stir in the spinach to wilt. Season to taste with salt and pepper. Top servings with pecans.

Chopped Kale Salad with Thai Peanut Dressing

Start to finish: 25 minutes
Serves 4

For the dressing:

¼ cup unsweetened natural creamy peanut butter (should contain only peanuts, with or without salt)

2 tablespoons unseasoned rice vinegar

2 tablespoons pineapple juice

2 tablespoons coconut aminos (like soy sauce, but made with coconut so it's soy- and gluten-free)

½ teaspoon toasted sesame oil

½ teaspoon grated fresh ginger

¼ teaspoon grated lime peel

1 to 2 tablespoons water, if needed

For the salad:

5 cups coarsely chopped baby kale

1½ cups shredded red cabbage

1 cup cooked shelled edamame

¾ cup coarsely shredded carrots

1 mango, peeled, pitted, and diced

1 small red bell pepper, seeded and diced

¼ small English cucumber, halved lengthwise and sliced

2 medium green onions, thinly sliced

¼ cup loosely packed chopped fresh cilantro, plus more for garnish if desired

½ cup roasted unsalted peanuts

1. For the dressing, in a small food processor or blender container, combine peanut butter, vinegar, pineapple juice, coconut aminos, sesame oil, ginger, and lime peel. Cover and process or blend until smooth. If necessary, add 1 to 2 tablespoons of water to make dressing desired consistency.

2. For the salad, place the kale in a large salad bowl. Drizzle with half the dressing. With clean hands, massage the kale for 2 to 4 minutes to tenderize it. Add the cabbage, edamame, carrots, mango, bell pepper, cucumber, green onions, and cilantro. Drizzle with remaining dressing.

3. Toss until combined. Sprinkle with peanuts. Garnish with additional cilantro, if desired.

Mango Tuna Salad–Stuffed Popovers

Start to finish: 30 minutes

Serves 6

For the popovers:

1 tablespoon ghee or coconut oil

4 large eggs

½ cup canned coconut milk

3 tablespoons coconut flour

¼ teaspoon fine sea salt

For the tuna salad:

½ cup Basic Homemade Mayonnaise (recipe follows) or compliant mayonnaise, such as mayo made with avocado oil

2 teaspoons fresh lime juice

2 (5-ounce) cans wild-caught albacore tuna, drained

1½ cups diced mango

¼ cup chopped red onion

½ cup diced jicama

3 tablespoons chopped fresh basil

Kosher salt and freshly ground black pepper

1. For the popovers, preheat the oven to 425°F. Place ½ teaspoon ghee in each of 6 popover cups or 2½-inch muffin cups. Place the popover or muffin pan in the oven while preparing the batter.

2. In a blender, combine the eggs, coconut milk, coconut flour, and salt. Cover and blend until well combined. Carefully remove the pan from oven. Fill the prepared cups half full of the batter. Bake for 20 to 25 minutes or until puffed and golden. Remove from the pan; cool on a wire rack.

3. Meanwhile, for the tuna salad, in a medium bowl stir together the mayonnaise and lime juice. Add the tuna, mango, red onion, jicama, and basil. Toss until combined. Season to taste with salt and pepper.

4. To serve, using a serrated knife, split the popovers lengthwise in half. Place the halves open on salad plates. Spoon and mound the tuna salad in the center of each half.

Basic Homemade Mayonnaise

In a blender, combine 1 large egg (at room temperature), ½ teaspoon dry mustard, ¼ teaspoon salt, 1 teaspoon fresh lemon juice, and 1 teaspoon apple cider vinegar. Cover; pulse to mix thoroughly. While the blender is running, slowly add 1 cup avocado oil or light-tasting olive oil through the feed tube until the mixture is emulsified. Store in an airtight container in the refrigerator for up to 1 week.

Quick Dal with Cauliflower Rice

Prep: 5 minutes

Cook: 15 minutes

Serves 3 to 4

1 tablespoon ghee

1 teaspoon minced fresh ginger

1 garlic clove, minced

1 teaspoon curry powder

½ teaspoon garam masala

1 (9-ounce) package steamed lentils

¾ cup chicken-based Basic Bone Broth (page 252) or purchased compliant chicken bone broth

¾ cup coconut milk

½ teaspoon kosher salt

1 plum tomato, seeded and diced

1 large handful baby spinach, coarsely chopped

Cooked cauliflower rice, for serving

1. In a medium pot, melt the ghee over medium heat. Add the ginger and garlic. Cook and stir for 1 minute. Add the curry powder and garam masala. Cook and stir until the spices are fragrant, 30 seconds to 1 minute.

2. Add the lentils, broth, coconut milk, and salt. Bring to a boil. Add the tomato. Reduce the heat and simmer until slightly reduced, for 3 to 4 minutes. Add the spinach and stir. Simmer until the spinach cooks down slightly, for 2 to 3 minutes.

3. Serve over the cauliflower rice.

Smoked Salmon Salad

Start to finish: 15 minutes
Serves 4

½ cup Basic Homemade Mayonnaise (page 202) or compliant mayonnaise, such as mayo made with avocado oil

2 tablespoons rice vinegar or fresh lemon juice

2 tablespoons chopped fresh dill

¼ teaspoon kosher salt

⅛ teaspoon freshly ground black pepper

1 (5-ounce) container mixed salad greens

1 English cucumber, thinly sliced

2 (4-ounce) pieces compliant (sugar-free) smoked salmon or leftover cooked salmon, flaked

½ small red onion, thinly sliced

2 hard-cooked eggs, cut into wedges

1 tablespoon drained capers

Chopped fresh dill or chives, for garnish (optional)

1. For the dressing, in a small bowl stir together the mayonnaise, vinegar, dill, salt, and pepper.

2. Smear some of the dressing on each plate. Top the dressing with the greens. Arrange the cucumber slices, salmon, onion, eggs, and capers on the greens. Garnish with additional dill or chives, if desired.

Sweet Potato BLTs

Start to finish: 30 minutes
Serves 4 (2 sandwiches each)

For the buns:

3 large roundish sweet potatoes, peeled (choose the ones that look the most bun-shaped)

2 tablespoons coconut oil

¼ teaspoon kosher salt

For the filling:

8 slices compliant (sugar-free) bacon

3 tablespoons compliant chipotle mayonnaise or Basic Homemade Mayonnaise (page 202) or compliant mayonnaise, such as mayonnaise made with avocado oil, plus a dash of chipotle chili powder

1 small tomato, cut into 8 slices

8 small lettuce leaves

1. For the buns, preheat oven to 400°F. Line two large baking sheets with parchment paper.

2. Wash the sweet potatoes; dry well with a clean kitchen towel. Cut sixteen ½-inch-thick potato slices from the widest portion of the sweet potatoes. In a large bowl, toss the sweet potato slices with coconut oil and salt. Place in a single layer on prepared baking sheets. Bake for 20 to 25 minutes or until tender yet firm enough to hold the sandwich fillings.

3. Meanwhile, in a large skillet, cook the bacon over medium heat for about 8 minutes or until nearly crisp. Transfer the bacon to paper towels to drain. Cut the slices crosswise in half.

4. To assemble the sandwiches, spread the mayonnaise on one side of each of the potato slices. Top half of the potato slices with two bacon slice halves, a tomato slice, and a lettuce leaf. Cover with remaining potato slices, mayonnaise sides down. If necessary, use sandwich picks to hold sandwiches together.

Waldorf Salad Wrap

Start to finish: 15 minutes
Serves 4

1 cup diced crisp apple

2 celery stalks, sliced

½ cup seedless grapes, halved or quartered

1 cup chopped leftover cooked chicken (optional)

½ cup chopped toasted pecans

¼ cup dried unsweetened tart cherries or cranberries

½ cup Basic Homemade Mayonnaise (page 202) or compliant mayonnaise, such as mayo made with avocado oil

1 tablespoon cider vinegar

1 to 2 tablespoons chopped fresh tarragon

½ teaspoon coarse salt

¼ teaspoon freshly ground black pepper

8 Bibb lettuce leaves

1. In a large bowl, stir together the apple, celery, grapes, chicken (if using), pecans, and cherries.

2. For the dressing, in a small bowl, stir together the mayonnaise, vinegar, tarragon, salt, and pepper.

3. Add the dressing to the salad; stir to coat. Spoon the salad onto the lettuce leaves.

Core4 Dinners

Breakfast-Anytime Nachos

Start to finish: 40 minutes

Serves 4

4 slices compliant (sugar-free) bacon, chopped into ½-inch pieces

2 medium sweet potatoes, peeled

1 red bell pepper, seeded and diced

Kosher salt and freshly ground black pepper

4 eggs

1 avocado, halved, pitted, peeled, and diced

2 green onions, chopped

1 jalapeño, seeded if desired, and sliced

Chopped fresh cilantro (optional)

Compliant salsa, for serving

1. Preheat the oven to 450°F. Place the bacon in a single layer on a 15×10-inch baking pan. Roast for 8 to 10 minutes or until the bacon is crisp. Use a slotted spoon to transfer the bacon to paper towels. Discard all but 2 tablespoons of the pan drippings.

2. Meanwhile, use a mandoline to slice the potatoes into ⅛-inch slices. Spread the potatoes in a single layer on the baking pan; turn to coat with the reserved bacon drippings. Sprinkle with the bell pepper. Season to taste with salt and pepper. Roast for 15 minutes or until the potatoes are tender and the edges are browned. Reduce the oven temperature to 400°F.

3. Carefully crack the eggs on top of the potatoes, being careful not to break the yolks. Bake for 8 to 10 minutes or until the whites are set.

4. Top the nachos with the bacon, avocado, green onions, jalapeño, and cilantro, if desired. Serve with salsa.

Cauliflower-Walnut Tacos

Prep: 15 minutes
Roast: 20 minutes
Serves 4

½ cup sun-dried tomatoes (not oil-packed)

2 cups cauliflower florets

1 cup walnut halves

¼ cup sunflower seeds

2 garlic cloves, minced

1 teaspoon ground cumin

2 teaspoons chili powder

½ teaspoon smoked paprika

½ teaspoon kosher salt

8 Bibb lettuce leaves

1 avocado, halved, pitted, and sliced, or 1 cup purchased compliant guacamole, for serving

Compliant salsa, for serving

Chopped fresh cilantro, for serving

1. Preheat the oven to 450°F. In a small bowl, combine the sun-dried tomatoes and hot water to cover. Let sit for 5 minutes; drain, reserving the soaking water.

2. In a food processor, combine the cauliflower, walnuts, sunflower seeds, drained sun-dried tomatoes, garlic, cumin, chili powder, paprika, and salt. Add 1 tablespoon of the reserved tomato water. Process until the mixture resembles small peas. Transfer to a large rimmed baking sheet. Bake for 20 minutes or until the cauliflower is tender and the mixture is browned.

3. Serve the taco filling in lettuce leaves; top with the avocado, salsa, and cilantro.

Ginger-Garlic Shrimp and Cabbage

Prep: 10 minutes
Roast: 20 minutes
Serves 4

4 medium carrots, sliced on an angle

1 large red bell pepper, seeded and coarsely chopped

1 tablespoon olive oil

Coarse salt and freshly ground black pepper

3 tablespoons coconut aminos

2 teaspoons toasted sesame oil

1 tablespoon grated or minced fresh ginger

3 garlic cloves, minced

1 pound medium shrimp, peeled and deveined

1 small head napa cabbage, cut into thin wedges

½ to 1 cup compliant kimchi, drained

Chopped green onions, for serving

Toasted sesame seeds, for serving

1. Preheat the oven to 400°F. Position a rack in the center of the oven. Line a rimmed baking sheet with parchment paper.

2. Place the carrot and bell pepper on the prepared pan. Drizzle with the olive oil and season lightly with salt and pepper; toss to coat. Roast for 10 minutes. Meanwhile, in a small bowl, stir together the coconut aminos, sesame oil, ginger, and garlic.

3. Push the carrots and bell pepper to one side of the pan; add the shrimp and cabbage. Season the vegetables and shrimp with salt and pepper to taste. Drizzle with the coconut amino mixture. Top the cabbage with the kimchi. Roast for 10 minutes or until the vegetables are crisp-tender and the shrimp are opaque.

4. Top servings with the green onions and sesame seeds.

Pan-Seared Salmon on Bitter Greens with Sweet Cherries

Prep: 20 minutes

Cook: 15 minutes

Serves 4

For the salmon:

4 (5-ounce) center-cut salmon fillets, each about 1 inch thick

1 teaspoon kosher salt

½ teaspoon coarse freshly ground black pepper

1 tablespoon olive oil

1 teaspoon ghee

For the salad:

3 tablespoons fresh orange juice

2 tablespoons extra-virgin olive oil

1 teaspoon white wine vinegar or apple cider vinegar

Kosher salt and freshly ground black pepper

2 small heads radicchio, cored and leaves slightly torn

1 cup loosely packed arugula

½ cup torn beet greens or Asian mustard greens

2 tablespoons chopped fresh flat-leaf parsley

1 cup fresh Bing or Rainier cherries, pitted and halved

1. For the salmon, season the salmon with the salt and pepper.

2. In a large cast-iron skillet, heat the oil and ghee over medium-high heat until shimmering. Place the salmon, skin side up, in the pan. Cook until golden brown on one side, about 4 minutes. Turn the salmon over with a spatula and cook until it feels firm to the touch, about 3 minutes more.

3. Meanwhile, for the salad, in a large bowl, whisk together the orange juice, oil, and vinegar until well blended. Season to taste with salt and pepper. Add the radicchio, arugula, beet greens, and parsley. Lightly toss until coated.

4. To serve, spoon the greens onto four plates. Top each with a salmon fillet. Sprinkle the cherries on top. Serve warm.

Pesto-Stuffed Chicken Breasts with Chunky Tomato Sauce

Prep: 30 minutes

Cook: 25 minutes

Serves 4

For the pesto and chicken:

2 cups lightly packed fresh basil leaves*

¼ cup pine nuts

2 large garlic cloves, coarsely chopped

2 teaspoons fresh lemon juice

¼ teaspoon kosher salt

1 teaspoon nutritional yeast (optional)

3 tablespoons olive oil

4 (6-ounce) boneless, skinless chicken breast halves

*NOTE: For spinach pesto, substitute 1½ cups lightly packed baby spinach plus ½ cup lightly packed fresh basil for the 2 cups basil.

For the sauce:

1 tablespoon olive oil

½ cup chopped leeks (white part only)

1 large garlic clove minced

1 (28-ounce) can whole peeled plum tomatoes, undrained, chopped

Kosher salt and freshly ground black pepper

¼ teaspoon compliant balsamic vinegar

1. For the pesto, in a food processor, combine the basil, pine nuts, garlic, lemon juice, salt, and nutritional yeast, if using. Cover and process until the basil is coarsely chopped. With the food processor running, add the oil in a thin stream just until mixture is smooth.

2. For the chicken, place each breast half between two pieces of plastic wrap. Using the flat side of a meat mallet, pound to ¼-inch thickness. Place one-fourth of the pesto mixture in the center of each chicken breast. Evenly spread the pesto to the edge of the chicken, leaving a ¼-inch border uncovered. Starting at the narrow end, roll up each breast jelly-roll style. If necessary, secure with wooden toothpicks. Place the rolled breasts, seam side down, on a plate.

3. For the sauce, in a large skillet heat olive oil over medium heat. Add the leeks. Cook and stir for 5 minutes or until nearly tender. Add the garlic and cook for 1 minute more or until leeks are tender. Add the undrained tomatoes and gently simmer for 5 minutes, stirring occasionally. Season to taste with salt and pepper. Stir in the balsamic vinegar. Add the stuffed chicken breasts. Cover and cook over medium heat for 15 to 20 minutes or until a thermometer registers 165°F.

4. To serve, if necessary, remove toothpicks. Serve whole or sliced with sauce spooned alongside.

Root Vegetable Curry

Prep: 15 minutes

Cook: 15 minutes

Serves 4

2½ cups compliant vegetable broth

¾ cup compliant coconut cream*

2 tablespoons compliant green or red curry paste

¼ teaspoon kosher salt

1 tablespoon coconut oil

1½ cups peeled and diced sweet potatoes

½ cup peeled and diced parsnips

¼ cup thinly slivered yellow onion

1 (15-ounce) can chickpeas, drained and rinsed

1 (12-ounce) package frozen riced cauliflower

¼ cup roasted unsalted cashews, coarsely chopped

2 tablespoons chopped fresh cilantro

1. In a medium bowl, whisk together the broth, coconut cream, curry paste, and salt.

2. In a large nonstick skillet, heat oil over medium heat. Add the sweet potatoes and parsnips. Cook for 3 minutes, stirring occasionally. Add the onion and cook 1 minute more. Add the broth mixture and chickpeas. Bring to a boil; reduce heat. Cover and simmer for 10 minutes or until the vegetables are tender, stirring occasionally.

3. Meanwhile, heat the riced cauliflower according to the package directions. Serve the curry over the riced cauliflower. Top with the cashews and cilantro.

*NOTE: This is a canned product and is thicker than coconut milk. Use only unsweetened varieties. The cream that rises to the top of a can of full-fat coconut milk is also coconut cream. If you can't find unsweetened coconut cream, you can use that.

Weeknight Beef Pho

Start to finish: 30 minutes

Serves 4

12 ounces organic grass-fed flank steak

2 tablespoons coconut oil

Kosher salt and freshly ground black pepper

5 cups beef-based Basic Bone Broth (page 252) or compliant purchased beef bone broth

2 teaspoons coconut aminos

2 teaspoons compliant fish sauce

1 tablespoon minced fresh ginger

2 medium carrots, cut into thin matchsticks or coarsely shredded

1 (10.7-ounce to 12-ounce) package zucchini noodles

¼ cup chopped green onion

1 fresh serrano or jalapeño pepper, sliced (optional)

½ cup chopped fresh mint, basil, and/or cilantro

1 lime, cut into wedges

1. If desired, partially freeze the beef for easier slicing, about 20 minutes. Cut the flank steak in half lengthwise and then thinly slice each half across the grain into strips. Cut the strips in half. In a 4-quart Dutch oven or large pot, melt the coconut oil over medium heat. Add the steak and lightly season with salt and pepper. Cook for 2 minutes or just until browned on both sides, stirring occasionally. Remove the steak from Dutch oven and set aside. Carefully add the broth, coconut aminos, fish sauce, and ginger. Bring the broth to a boil over medium-high heat.

2. Add the carrots and zucchini noodles to the broth. Cook for 2 minutes or until the noodles are crisp-tender.

3. Return the steak to the broth. Ladle the pho into bowls and top servings with green onion, serrano (if using), and fresh herbs. Serve with lime wedges.

Core4 Snacks

....

Buffalo Chicken Dip

Prep: 10 minutes
Bake: 20 minutes
Serves 8

1 tablespoon ghee

½ cup chopped yellow onion

2 garlic cloves, minced

⅔ cup Basic Homemade Mayonnaise (page 202) or compliant mayonnaise, such as mayo made with avocado oil

1 (5.4-ounce) can unsweetened coconut cream* (about ⅔ cup)

1 tablespoon compliant Dijon mustard

¼ teaspoon smoked paprika

1 teaspoon garlic powder

½ teaspoon onion powder

½ teaspoon sea salt

¼ cup compliant hot sauce

1 tablespoon fresh lemon juice

2½ to 3 cups shredded cooked chicken

Sliced fresh vegetables, such as celery, zucchini, carrots, and/or red, orange, or yellow bell peppers, for serving

1. Preheat the oven to 350°F. In a large skillet, melt the ghee over medium heat. Add the onion and garlic; cook for 4 to 5 minutes or until the onion is softened.

2. Meanwhile, in a large bowl, stir together the mayonnaise, coconut cream, mustard, paprika, garlic powder, onion powder, salt, hot sauce, and lemon juice. Stir in the chicken. Stir in the cooked onion and garlic. Spoon into a 2-quart baking dish.

*NOTE: This is a canned product and is thicker than coconut milk. Use only unsweetened varieties. The cream that rises to the top of a can of full-fat coconut milk is also coconut cream. If you can't find unsweetened coconut cream, you can use that.

3. Bake, uncovered, for 20 minutes or until heated through and the edges are bubbling.

4. Serve the dip with the sliced vegetables.

Cauliflower-Nut Flatbreads

Prep: 10 minutes

Bake: 15 minutes

Serves 6 (4 flatbreads each)

4 cups small cauliflower florets

1 large egg

2 tablespoons olive oil

½ cup almond meal

½ teaspoon kosher salt

⅛ teaspoon cayenne pepper

1 tablespoon nutritional yeast

1. Preheat the oven to 425°F. Line two baking sheets with parchment paper.

2. Place the cauliflower in a food processor. Cover and pulse until the cauliflower is finely chopped but not pureed. Add the egg, oil, almond meal, salt, cayenne, and nutritional yeast. Cover and process just until well combined.

3. Spoon 2 tablespoons of the mixture onto the prepared baking sheet. Using the back of a spoon, spread it to ⅛-inch thickness. Repeat with the remaining cauliflower mixture.

4. Bake for 10 to 15 minutes or until the tops are golden. Using a wide spatula, turn the breads over. Bake for 2 to 3 minutes or until golden.

5. Transfer the breads to a wire rack. Eat warm or at room temperature.

Chili-Spiced Nuts and Cranberries

Start to finish: 25 minutes

Makes 2½ cups (¼ cup per serving)

1 teaspoon chili powder

¾ teaspoon coarse sea salt

¼ teaspoon garlic powder

¼ teaspoon freshly ground black
 pepper

⅛ teaspoon ground cumin

1 tablespoon olive or avocado oil

1 cup raw whole almonds

½ cup raw whole cashews or
 macadamia nuts

½ cup raw pecan halves

¼ cup raw pepitas (shelled
 pumpkin seeds)

⅓ cup fruit-juice-sweetened
 dried cranberries or cherries

1. Preheat the oven to 325°F. Line a large rimmed baking sheet with parchment paper.

2. In a medium bowl, combine the chili powder, salt, garlic powder, pepper, and cumin. Stir in the oil until well combined. Add the almonds, cashews, pecans, and pepitas; toss until evenly coated with the oil mixture. Spread in a single layer on the prepared baking sheet.

3. Bake for 12 to 15 minutes or until the nuts are lightly toasted, stirring halfway through baking.

4. Remove from the oven. Add the cranberries; stir until combined. Let stand until cooled. Store in an airtight container at room temperature for up to 1 week.

Chocolate, Coconut, and Hemp Energy Balls

Prep: 10 minutes

Freeze: 20 minutes

Makes 12

8 Medjool dates,* pitted

¼ cup hemp hearts

¼ cup unsweetened cocoa
 powder

2 tablespoons unsweetened
shredded coconut

1 tablespoon coconut oil, melted

¼ teaspoon vanilla extract

¼ teaspoon sea salt

2 tablespoons finely chopped
unsweetened dark chocolate

1. In a food processor, pulse the dates until a ball forms. Add the
hemp hearts, cocoa powder, coconut, coconut oil, vanilla, salt, and
chocolate. Process until well combined and almost smooth.
The dough will be sticky; if not moist enough to form a ball,
add 1 teaspoon of water at a time and pulse to combine. If too wet,
add additional hemp hearts 1 teaspoon at a time and pulse to
combine.

2. Line a baking sheet or plate with parchment paper. Use a 1-inch
scoop or your hands, wetted if necessary, to shape the dough into
12 balls. Place the baking sheet in the freezer for 20 minutes or until
firm. Store the leftovers in an airtight container in the refrigerator
for up to 1 week, or freeze for up to 1 month.

*NOTE: If the dates are not moist, soak them in a bowl of hot water to cover for
10 minutes. Drain the water and pat dry with paper towels.

Crunchy Roasted Chickpeas

Prep: 10 minutes
Cook: 1 hour 30 minutes
Serves 8

2 (15-ounce) cans chickpeas,
drained and rinsed

2 tablespoons olive oil

1 teaspoon kosher salt

2 teaspoons desired spice or spice
blend, such as curry powder,
chili powder, garam masala,
smoked paprika, or jerk
seasoning (optional)

1. Preheat the oven to 350°F. Place the rinsed chickpeas in a salad
spinner and spin a few times to get most of the water off. Turn the

chickpeas onto a paper-towel-lined rimmed baking pan. Top with another layer of paper towels and roll to remove any remaining dampness. The chickpeas should look matte and feel completely dry.

2. Remove the paper towels from the baking pan. Spread the chickpeas out onto the baking pan. Drizzle with the oil and sprinkle with the salt. Toss to evenly coat.

3. Roast the chickpeas for 30 minutes. Sprinkle with desired spice blend, if using, and toss to coat evenly. Turn the oven off and leave the chickpeas in the oven to dry and crisp up for about 1 hour.

4. Let cool completely before storing in a tightly sealed container.

Guacamole-Stuffed Baby Bells

Start to finish: 30 minutes
Serves 6 (2 halves each)

6 red, yellow, and/or orange mini bell peppers

1 very ripe Hass avocado

1 tablespoon finely chopped green onion

1 tablespoon fresh lime juice

2 teaspoons minced fresh cilantro

1 teaspoon minced jalapeño

1 garlic clove, minced

¼ teaspoon sea salt

3 slices compliant bacon, cooked until crisp and crumbled

6 grape tomatoes, sliced

1. Cut the peppers lengthwise in half. Carefully remove the seeds and white membranes.

2. Cut the avocado lengthwise in half and remove the pit. Using a spoon, scoop the pulp into a bowl. Using a fork, mash the pulp until smooth. Stir in the green onion, lime juice, cilantro, jalapeño, garlic, and salt.

3. Fill each pepper half with 2 to 3 teaspoons of the avocado mixture. Top with the crumbled bacon and tomato slices.

Zucchini Hummus Cucumber Sushi Rolls

Start to finish: 15 minutes

Serves 4 to 5

2 small zucchini, peeled and coarsely chopped

1 garlic clove, halved

2 tablespoons fresh lemon juice

3 tablespoons tahini

1 tablespoon extra-virgin olive oil

½ teaspoon ground cumin

⅛ teaspoon smoked or regular paprika

¼ teaspoon kosher salt

1 English cucumber

Lemon zest, for garnish (optional)

1. In a food processor, combine the zucchini, garlic, lemon juice, tahini, olive oil, cumin, paprika, and salt. Process until smooth and creamy.

2. Using a Y vegetable peeler or mandoline set on the thinnest setting, slice the cucumber into thin slices, discarding the first and the last slice, which is mostly the cucumber skin. (If using a regular cucumber, peel, then slice just down to the seeds on two sides.)

3. Spoon about 2 teaspoons of the hummus down the center of each cucumber slice; gently roll up. Garnish with the lemon zest, if desired.

NOTE: To make this recipe Elimin8-friendly, use compliant guacamole instead of the zucchini hummus.

Breakfast Steaks with Sweet Potato Hash Browns

Prep: 15 minutes

Cook: 15 minutes

Serves 2

1 medium sweet potato, peeled and shredded

2 green onions, minced

6 tablespoons olive oil, divided

Kosher salt and coarse freshly ground black pepper

2 tablespoons compliant prepared horseradish

2 tablespoons Egg-Free Mayonnaise (page 230)

1 teaspoon finely chopped fresh chives

½ teaspoon lemon zest

½ teaspoon kosher salt

⅛ teaspoon coarse freshly ground black pepper

2 (5-ounce) rib-eye steaks, ½ inch thick each

1. In a medium bowl, combine the sweet potato and green onion. Drizzle with 3 tablespoons of the oil and season with salt and pepper to taste; toss to combine. Preheat the oven to 250°F.

2. Heat a large cast-iron skillet over medium heat. Add 2 tablespoons of the oil to the hot skillet. Add the potatoes to the skillet,* leaving a ½-inch border around the edge (potatoes will flatten as they cook). Cook for 8 to 10 minutes, until golden brown and crisp on the bottom. Use a large spatula to turn the hash browns, adding additional olive oil if needed. Cook for 4 to 5 minutes more or until golden brown and crisp on the bottom. Remove from the skillet and keep warm on a large rimmed baking pan in the oven.

*NOTE: Test the griddle with a few strands of sweet potato to make sure it's hot; if they sizzle, the pan is ready.

3. Meanwhile, for the horseradish sauce, in a small bowl, combine the horseradish, mayonnaise, chives, lemon zest, salt, and pepper.

4. Heat the remaining 1 tablespoon oil in the skillet over medium-high heat. When the skillet is hot, add the steaks and cook for 2 minutes on each side (145°F for medium).

5. Spread the horseradish sauce on the steaks. Serve the steaks with the hash browns.

Brussels Sprouts, Bacon, Apple, and Salmon Skillet

Start to finish: 15 minutes

Serves 2

3 slices compliant bacon

1 large shallot, thinly sliced

1 (9- to 10-ounce) bag shredded Brussels sprouts

½ small apple, peeled, cored, and coarsely shredded

1 to 1½ cups cooked flaked salmon

¼ teaspoon kosher salt

¼ teaspoon coarse freshly ground black pepper

1 teaspoon coconut aminos

½ ripe avocado, halved, pitted, peeled, and diced

1 teaspoon lemon zest

Chopped fresh dill, basil, or flat-leaf parsley

1. In a large skillet, cook the bacon over medium heat for 5 to 8 minutes or until crisp, turning once. Transfer the bacon to paper towels to drain; crumble when cool. Remove all but 1 tablespoon of the bacon fat from the skillet.

2. Add the shallot to the hot skillet; cook for 3 to 4 minutes or until softened and starting to get crispy. Stir in the Brussels sprouts. Cook, covered, for 2 minutes. Uncover and cook for 3 minutes or until crisp-tender, stirring occasionally.

3. Stir in the apple and salmon; season with salt, pepper, and coconut aminos. Cook for 2 to 3 minutes or until the salmon and apple are heated through.

4. Top servings with the crumbled bacon, avocado, lemon zest, and dill.

Herb-Crusted Cauliflower Steaks with Mushroom-Onion Scramble

Prep: 20 minutes

Roast: 30 minutes

Serves 2

1 (2-pound) head cauliflower, leaves removed, core intact

2 tablespoons olive oil, divided

¼ teaspoon coarse sea salt

¼ teaspoon coarse freshly ground black pepper

½ cup chopped yellow onion

1 (5-ounce) package sliced cremini mushrooms

1 garlic clove, minced

¼ cup chopped fresh flat-leaf parsley

2 tablespoons finely chopped unsulfured dried apricots

2 teaspoons orange zest

1. Preheat the oven to 425°F. Line a rimmed baking sheet with foil. Starting from the top, use a large knife to slice two 1-inch-thick slices from the cauliflower. (Reserve the remaining cauliflower for another use.) Place the slices on the prepared baking sheet; brush both sides with 1 tablespoon of the oil; sprinkle with the salt and pepper. Roast the cauliflower for 15 minutes; carefully turn. Roast for 10 to 15 minutes more or until tender.

2. Meanwhile, in a large skillet, heat the remaining 1 tablespoon oil over medium heat. Add the onion and cook for 3 to 4 minutes or until softened, stirring occasionally. Add the mushrooms and garlic; cook for 4 to 5 minutes or until the mushrooms have released their liquid and are beginning to brown, stirring

frequently (add additional olive oil, if necessary). Season to taste with additional salt.

3. In a small bowl, combine the parsley, apricots, and orange zest. If desired, lightly drizzle the cauliflower with additional olive oil. Serve the mushroom-onion scramble alongside the cauliflower and sprinkle with the parsley mixture.

Power Greens Smoothie

Start to finish: 5 minutes
Serves 2

1 small banana, cut into chunks

⅓ cup canned full-fat coconut milk

1 cup water

1 cup frozen mango chunks

½ cup frozen peach slices

½-inch-thick sliced peeled fresh ginger

¼ teaspoon ground turmeric

½ (5-ounce) package mixed power greens

1. In a blender, combine the banana, coconut milk, water, mango chunks, peach slices, ginger, turmeric, and greens. Blend until smooth.

2. Pour into two glasses; serve immediately.

Sausage-Stuffed Apples

Prep: 25 minutes
Bake: 35 minutes
Serves 4

2 tablespoons ghee, divided, plus additional for greasing baking dish

4 medium Braeburn or Honeycrisp apples

¾ cup plus 3 tablespoons 100% fresh-pressed, pasteurized apple cider

1½ teaspoons kosher salt, divided

1 teaspoon garlic powder

1 teaspoon onion powder

1 teaspoon dried ground sage

½ teaspoon dried thyme leaves

¼ teaspoon freshly ground black pepper

1 pound ground lean pork or turkey

1½ teaspoons arrowroot powder

1 (10-ounce) package frozen riced butternut squash, cooked according to package directions, for serving

1. Preheat the oven to 425°F. Lightly grease a 13×9-inch baking dish with a small amount of ghee.

2. Cut the apples lengthwise in half. Cut a very thin slice off the uncut sides so the apples lie flat. Using a melon baller, core and discard the seeds. Scoop out the insides, leaving ¼- to ½-inch-thick shells. Finely chop the apple pulp.

3. In a small skillet, melt 1 tablespoon of the ghee over medium heat. Add the apple pulp. Cook for 3 to 5 minutes or until it softens, stirring occasionally. Remove from heat; transfer to a large bowl. Stir in 1 tablespoon of the apple cider, 1 teaspoon of the salt, garlic powder, onion powder, sage, thyme, and pepper. Let mixture cool.

4. Add the pork to the apple mixture in bowl. Gently combine, being careful not to overmix. Loosely stuff the sausage mixture into the apple shells. Place the stuffed apples in the prepared baking dish. Bake, uncovered, for 35 to 40 minutes or until a thermometer inserted near the center of the filling registers 160°F for pork or 165° for turkey.

5. Meanwhile, for the sauce, in a small saucepan whisk together 2 tablespoons of the apple cider and arrowroot until well blended. Whisk in the ¾ cup apple cider. Cook and stir over medium heat until bubbly. Reduce heat; cook and stir 1 minute.

6. To serve, toss the cooked butternut squash with the remaining 1 tablespoon ghee and ½ teaspoon salt. Divide among four serving plates. Place stuffed apples on the bed of squash. Drizzle with sauce.

Shrimp, Bacon, and Okra with Garlicky Cauliflower Grits

Start to finish: 30 minutes

Serves 4

For the grits:

- 3 tablespoons ghee
- 2 garlic cloves, minced
- 1 teaspoon coconut aminos
- ½ cup chicken-based Basic Bone Broth (page 252) or purchased compliant chicken bone broth
- 2 (12-ounce) packages frozen riced cauliflower
- 1 teaspoon coarse salt
- 1 teaspoon coarse freshly ground black pepper

For the shrimp:

- 2 slices compliant bacon
- 1 tablespoon ghee
- ¾ cup coarsely chopped yellow onion
- ¾ teaspoon coarse salt
- ¾ teaspoon coarse freshly ground pepper
- 1 teaspoon dried oregano, crushed
- ½ teaspoon garlic powder
- 1 pound fresh okra, trimmed and sliced, or 1 (12-ounce) bag frozen chopped okra
- 1 pound medium shrimp, peeled and deveined
- 1 tablespoon fresh lemon juice
- Chopped fresh flat-leaf parsley, for garnish (optional)

1. For the grits, in a large skillet, melt the ghee over medium heat. Add the garlic and cook for 30 seconds. Stir in the coconut aminos, broth, and cauliflower; season with the salt and pepper. Cook, stirring frequently, for 5 minutes or until the cauliflower is tender. If desired, use an immersion blender to blend the cauliflower until almost smooth. Cover and keep warm.

2. Meanwhile, for the shrimp, in another large skillet, cook the bacon over medium heat until crisp. Transfer to a paper-towel-lined plate to drain. Crumble the bacon when cooled. Remove all but

1 tablespoon of the drippings from the skillet. Add the ghee to the drippings. Add the onion and cook for 8 to 10 minutes or until tender, stirring occasionally.

3. In a small bowl, stir together the salt and pepper, oregano, and garlic powder. Add the okra to the onions; sprinkle with the seasoning. Raise the heat to medium-high. Cook for 3 minutes, stirring frequently. Add the shrimp; cook for 3 minutes more or until the shrimp are opaque and the okra is crisp-tender, stirring frequently. Stir in the lemon juice.

4. Divide the grits among four plates. Top with the shrimp mixture. Garnish with parsley, if desired.

Sweet Potato–Date Smoothie

Start to finish: 5 minutes
Serves 1

½ cup frozen banana slices*

⅓ cup coarsely shredded carrot

⅓ cup apple juice

2 to 3 ice cubes

2 Medjool dates, pitted and chopped

⅔ cup cooked, mashed, and cooled sweet potato

Pinch ground cinnamon

1. In a blender container, combine the banana slices, shredded carrot, apple juice, ice cubes, and dates. Cover and blend until nearly smooth.

2. Add the sweet potato. Cover and blend until smooth. Pour into a glass. Sprinkle with cinnamon.

*NOTE: To keep the frozen banana slices on hand for smoothies, peel some bananas and cut them into ½-inch slices. Toss the banana slices in a small amount of orange juice to prevent them from turning brown. Drain the banana slices and freeze in a single layer on a parchment-paper-lined baking sheet. When frozen, store the banana slices in a tightly covered freezer container or a resealable plastic freezer bag.

Elimin8 Lunches

Cauliflower-Broccoli Tabbouleh

Prep: 10 minutes

Cool: 30 minutes

Serves 4

3 tablespoons olive oil, plus additional for serving

2 (10- or 12-ounce) packages frozen riced cauliflower-broccoli or about 5 cups riced cauliflower

1 teaspoon kosher salt, divided

3 tablespoons fresh lemon juice

¼ cup coarsely chopped pitted Kalamata olives

1 medium English cucumber, chopped

2 green onions, thinly sliced

¼ cup chopped fresh mint

½ cup chopped fresh curly-leaf parsley

Lemon wedges (optional)

1. In a large skillet, heat the oil over medium-high heat. Add the cauliflower and ½ teaspoon of the salt. Cook for 5 minutes or until crisp-tender, stirring occasionally. Spread the cauliflower on a large piece of foil or parchment paper to cool.*

2. In a large bowl, stir together the remaining ½ teaspoon salt and the lemon juice. Add the cooled cauliflower, olives, cucumber, green onions, mint, and parsley; gently stir to combine.

3. Serve with lemon wedges, if desired, and drizzle with the additional olive oil.

*NOTE: The cauliflower can be prepared the day before; cover and refrigerate until ready to use.

Chicken Zoodle Soup

Start to finish: 30 minutes

Serves 4

1 pound boneless, skinless chicken breast halves

3 tablespoons olive oil, divided

1 medium yellow onion, chopped

2 celery stalks, diced

1 medium carrot, diced

4 cups chicken-based Basic Bone Broth (page 252) or purchased compliant chicken bone broth

2 cups water

½ teaspoon dried thyme

½ teaspoon kosher salt

¼ teaspoon freshly ground black pepper

2 cups packaged zucchini noodles

2 tablespoons finely chopped fresh parsley

1. Pat moisture from the chicken with paper towels. In a large saucepan, heat 2 tablespoons of the oil over medium-high heat. Add the chicken and cook for 6 to 8 minutes or until browned, turning once. (The chicken will not be cooked through at this point.) Transfer the chicken to a cutting board and dice; set aside.

2. Heat the remaining 1 tablespoon oil in the same saucepan over medium heat. Add the onion, celery, and carrot. Cook and stir for 4 minutes or until the onion begins to soften. Add the broth, water, thyme, salt, and pepper. Bring to boil. Add the chicken. Cover and simmer for 6 to 8 minutes or until the chicken is cooked through. Add the zucchini noodles. Cover and simmer for 1 to 2 minutes or until the noodles are crisp-tender. Stir in the parsley.

Lemony Fish Soup with Herbs and Greens

Prep: 10 minutes

Cook: 10 minutes

Serves 2

3 cups chicken-based Basic Bone Broth (page 252) or purchased compliant chicken bone broth

1 teaspoon lemon zest

¼ teaspoon kosher salt

8 ounces cod fillets (or other firm white fish)

½ cup riced cauliflower

2 teaspoons fresh lemon juice

2 cups baby arugula, stems removed

½ cup finely shredded carrot

2 tablespoons very thinly sliced fresh mint leaves

1 scallion, thinly sliced (white and green parts)

1. In a medium pot, combine the broth and lemon zest. Bring the broth to a simmer. Reduce the heat so the broth is steaming but not simmering. Add the salt, fish, and riced cauliflower and cook until the fish and cauliflower are just tender, for about 5 minutes. Remove the fish from the broth and break into bite-sized chunks. Stir the lemon juice into the broth.

2. Divide the broth between two bowls. Top with the fish, arugula, carrot, mint, and scallions.

Salmon, Beet, and Shaved Fennel Salad

Start to finish: 15 minutes

Serves 4

1 (5-ounce) container mixed spring greens

1 fennel bulb, trimmed, cored, and shaved

1 (8-ounce) package refrigerated cooked whole baby beets, chopped

12 ounces cooked salmon, flaked

¼ cup extra-virgin olive oil or avocado oil

¼ cup fresh orange juice

2 tablespoons compliant balsamic vinegar

1 tablespoon minced shallot

¼ teaspoon kosher salt

¼ teaspoon coarse freshly ground black pepper

1. Arrange the greens on a serving platter or individual plates. Top with the fennel, beets, and salmon.

2. In a small bowl, whisk together the oil, orange juice, vinegar, shallot, salt, and pepper. Pour some of the dressing over salad(s).

3. Cover and refrigerate any leftover dressing for another use.

Shrimp Cakes with Creamy Dilled Slaw

Start to finish: 30 minutes
Serves 2

For the slaw:

½ cup Egg-Free Mayonnaise (page 230)

1 tablespoon apple cider vinegar

½ teaspoon dried dill

½ teaspoon kosher salt

Freshly ground black pepper

4 cups preshredded coleslaw mix (cabbage and carrot)

1 green onion, sliced

For the shrimp cakes:

8 ounces raw shrimp, peeled (tails removed) and deveined

2 tablespoons arrowroot powder

2 tablespoons finely diced red onion

2 tablespoons finely diced celery

1 tablespoon chopped fresh parsley

2 tablespoons Egg-Free Mayonnaise (page 230)

1 tablespoon fresh lemon juice

¼ teaspoon kosher salt, plus more as needed

¼ teaspoon garlic powder

Freshly ground black pepper

½ cup coconut flour

2 tablespoons ghee

Lemon wedges, for serving (optional)

1. For the slaw, in a small bowl combine the mayonnaise, vinegar, dillweed, salt, and pepper to taste. Place coleslaw and green onion in a medium bowl. Drizzle with the dressing. Toss to combine. Refrigerate while you make the shrimp cakes.

2. For the shrimp cakes, pat the shrimp dry with a paper towel and place in a food processor fitted with a metal blade. Pulse until the shrimp are finely chopped. Transfer to a medium bowl and add the arrowroot powder, onion, celery, parsley, mayonnaise, lemon juice, salt, garlic powder, and pepper to taste. Stir gently to combine.

3. On a small plate, combine the coconut flour with ⅛ teaspoon each of salt and pepper. Using a ⅓-cup measuring cup, scoop the shrimp mixture onto a separate plate. Using your hands, form the mixture into a patty. Dredge the patty in the coconut flour, set aside on a plate, then repeat with remaining mixture (you should end up with 4 patties).

4. In a large skillet, melt the ghee over medium-high heat. When hot, add the patties to the pan. Cook for 3 minutes, then carefully flip and cook for an additional 2 to 3 minutes.

5. Serve the shrimp cakes with the slaw and lemon wedges, if desired.

Egg-Free Mayonnaise

In a blender or food processor, combine the flesh of 1 medium avocado, ¼ cup olive oil, 1 tablespoon coconut butter, 1 tablespoon apple cider vinegar or fresh lemon juice, ¼ teaspoon garlic powder, and ¼ teaspoon salt. Cover and blend on high until smooth. Store in an airtight container in the refrigerator for up to 1 week. Stir before using.

Steak and Carrot Noodle Bowl with Chimichurri Sauce

Start to finish: 30 minutes

Serves 4

For the chimichurri sauce:

1 cup packed fresh flat-leaf parsley

2 tablespoons fresh oregano leaves

4 garlic cloves, peeled

3 tablespoons red wine vinegar

1 tablespoon fresh lemon juice

½ teaspoon kosher salt

½ cup extra-virgin olive oil

For the noodle bowl:

1 pound organic grass-fed flank steak

½ teaspoon kosher salt, plus more as needed

¼ teaspoon freshly ground black pepper, plus more as needed

1 tablespoon olive oil

1 (12-ounce) package frozen carrot noodles

4 cups baby arugula or spinach

1. For the chimichurri sauce, in a food processor, combine the parsley, oregano, and garlic; process until finely chopped. Add the vinegar, lemon juice, salt, and oil; pulse to combine.

2. Preheat the broiler. Position the oven rack 4 to 5 inches from the heat source.

3. For the noodle bowl, score both sides of the steak in a diamond pattern by making shallow diagonal cuts at 1-inch intervals. Season the steak with salt and pepper. Place steak on the unheated rack of a broiler pan. Broil for 13 to 16 minutes for medium (145°F), turning once halfway through. Transfer the steak to a cutting board. Tent with foil; let stand for 5 minutes. Thinly slice the steak across the grain, then cut into bite-sized pieces.

4. Meanwhile, heat the oil in a large skillet over medium heat. Add carrot noodles to the skillet. Cook 6 to 8 minutes or until tender, tossing frequently. Turn off the heat. Add arugula; toss to wilt. Season to taste with salt and pepper.

5. Divide the carrot noodles among shallow serving bowls; top with the steak and drizzle with the chimichurri sauce.

Veggie-Avocado Mash Coconut Wraps

Start to finish: 10 minutes

Serves 2

1 small ripe avocado, peeled, pitted, and cut into chunks

1 tablespoon fresh lemon juice

¼ teaspoon kosher salt

¼ teaspoon ground cumin

1 cup leftover roasted vegetables (such as cauliflower, broccoli, beets, onion, Brussels sprouts, sweet potatoes, or carrots)

2 compliant coconut wraps

Microgreens

1. In a medium bowl, combine the avocado, lemon juice, salt, and cumin. Mash with a fork until ingredients are well combined.

2. If desired, warm the vegetables in the microwave for 30 to 45 seconds.

3. Spread 2 to 3 tablespoons of the avocado mash* on each coconut wrap. Mound half of the vegetables down the center. Top with microgreens and serve.

*NOTE: Refrigerate the remaining mash and use as a dip or spread.

Elimin8 Dinners

Buttery Garlic-Tarragon Pan-Seared Scallops with Shaved Asparagus Salad

Start to finish: 20 minutes

Serves 4

For the salad:

2 tablespoons extra-virgin olive oil

4 teaspoons fresh lemon juice

2 teaspoons finely chopped shallot

⅛ teaspoon kosher salt

⅛ teaspoon freshly ground black pepper

1 pound asparagus, trimmed

For the scallops:

1 pound fresh or frozen sea scallops, thawed

½ teaspoon kosher salt

¼ teaspoon freshly ground black pepper

1 tablespoon olive oil

3 tablespoons ghee, divided

2 garlic cloves, thinly sliced

1 tablespoon fresh lemon juice

4 teaspoons chopped fresh tarragon leaves

1. For the salad, in a medium bowl, whisk together the olive oil, lemon juice, shallot, salt, and pepper. Use a vegetable peeler to shave the asparagus into long, thin strips. Place the strips and any tips that fall off in the bowl with the dressing; toss to combine.

2. For the scallops, pat scallops dry with paper towels. Sprinkle with salt and pepper. In a large heavy skillet, heat the oil and 1 tablespoon of the ghee over medium-high heat. Add the scallops; cook for 3 minutes or until golden brown on the bottom. Turn and cook for 2 to 3 minutes or until golden brown on the exterior and barely opaque. Transfer the scallops to a large plate. Reduce the heat to medium.

3. Add the remaining 2 tablespoons ghee to the hot skillet. Add the garlic and lemon juice. Cook for 1 to 2 minutes or until the garlic is fragrant and golden. Stir in the tarragon. Pour the garlic-butter sauce over scallops. Serve with the asparagus salad.

Chicken and Vegetable Lo Mein

Start to finish: 30 minutes

Serves 4

1 (2½- to 3-pound) spaghetti squash, halved, seeds removed

¼ cup coconut aminos

2 tablespoons apple cider vinegar

1 tablespoon pineapple juice

4 tablespoons coconut oil, divided

1 pound boneless, skinless chicken breasts or thighs, cut into 1-inch pieces

½ teaspoon kosher salt

¼ teaspoon coarse freshly ground black pepper

3 garlic cloves, minced

1 tablespoon grated fresh ginger

1 cup chopped yellow onion

2 (5-ounce) packages sliced shiitake mushrooms

1 cup thinly sliced celery

2 heads baby bok choy, thinly sliced

2 green onions, sliced

¼ cup packed chopped fresh cilantro

1. Place the spaghetti squash halves (one at a time if necessary) cut side down in a microwave-safe glass or ceramic baking dish. Fill the dish with about 1 inch of water. Microwave on high for 15 minutes or until tender. Transfer the dish to a wire rack and let the squash cool slightly. Use a fork to scrape the strands of squash from the inside (you should get about 6 cups).

2. In a small bowl, mix together coconut aminos, vinegar, and pineapple juice. Set the sauce aside.

3. In an extra-large skillet, melt 2 tablespoons of the coconut oil over medium-high heat. Add the chicken and cook, without stirring, for 2 minutes or until opaque. Stir; season with salt and pepper. Stir in the garlic and ginger. Cook for 3 minutes more or until cooked through. Transfer the chicken to a bowl.

4. In the same skillet, melt the remaining 2 tablespoons coconut oil over medium-high heat. Add the onion and cook for 2 minutes to soften, stirring occasionally. Add the mushrooms, celery, and bok choy. Cook for 3 to 4 minutes or until vegetables are crisp-tender, stirring frequently.

5. Return the chicken to the skillet; stir in the sauce. Cook just until heated through. Serve over the spaghetti squash. Top each serving with green onions and cilantro.

Creamy Coconut-Ginger Squash Soup

Start to finish: 30 minutes

Serves 4

2 tablespoons ghee

1 cup coarsely chopped yellow
onion

1 ripe pear, such as Bartlett,
peeled, halved, cored, and
coarsely chopped

2 (16-ounce) bags frozen
butternut squash (4 cups)

1 tablespoon grated fresh ginger

1 teaspoon ground turmeric

⅛ teaspoon ground cloves

1 teaspoon kosher salt

¼ teaspoon coarse freshly ground
black pepper

1 (13- to 14-ounce) can
unsweetened coconut milk

2 cups chicken-based Basic
Bone Broth (page 252) or
purchased compliant chicken
bone broth

Crumbled cooked bacon or
Prosciutto Chips (page 244),
(optional)

1. In a Dutch oven, melt the ghee over medium heat. Add the onion
   and cook, stirring occasionally, for 8 to 10 minutes or until tender
   and caramelized. Add the pear and squash; cook until the squash is
   lightly browned and the pear is tender. Stir in the ginger, turmeric,
   cloves, salt, pepper, coconut milk, and broth. Cook, stirring
   frequently, until heated through.

2. Using an immersion blender, carefully blend the soup until
   completely smooth. (Or let the soup cool slightly, then carefully
   transfer it in batches to a food processor or blender; process or blend
   until completely smooth.) If the soup is too thick, add water, 2
   tablespoons at a time, until desired consistency is reached.

3. Top each serving with crumbled bacon or Prosciutto Chips, if
   desired.

Jicama Fish Tacos

Prep: 30 minutes

Cook: 4 to 6 minutes per ½ inch thickness

Serves 4 (4 tacos each)

For the fish:

1 pound cod fillets

¼ cup avocado oil

3 tablespoons finely chopped shallot or red onion

1 garlic clove, minced

1 teaspoon lime zest

2 tablespoons fresh lime juice

2 tablespoons fresh orange juice

1 teaspoon dried oregano

¼ teaspoon sea salt

⅛ teaspoon freshly ground black pepper

For the tacos:

1 large jicama, peeled

Shredded romaine lettuce

Toppings: Diced mango, diced cucumbers, diced avocado, sliced radishes, chopped red onion, and/or chopped fresh cilantro

Lime wedges

1. For the fish, preheat a grill to medium-high heat. Measure the thickness of the fish fillets. Place the fish in a large resealable plastic bag. In a small bowl, combine the oil, shallot, garlic, lime zest and juice, orange juice, oregano, salt, and pepper. Pour the marinade over the fish; close the bag to seal. Turn the bag to evenly coat the fish. Marinate at room temperature for 15 minutes.

2. Meanwhile, for the tacos, cut the jicama crosswise in half. Trim the edges, keeping the round shape, to about 4 inches in diameter or until the jicama will fit in a mandoline. Place the mandoline on its thinnest setting or use the blade that makes the thinnest slices, and cut the jicama to make 16 large round slices. If you don't have a mandoline, use a knife

to make very thin slices—they should be thin enough to bend and wrap around the fillings. Cover and set the jicama slices aside. Cover and refrigerate the remaining jicama; reserve for another use.

3. Remove the fish from the marinade. Grill the fish, uncovered, directly over heat for 4 to 6 minutes per ½-inch thickness or until the fish flakes easily, turning the fish over halfway through grilling. Transfer the fish to a platter and flake into large pieces.

4. To assemble the tacos, top each jicama slice with lettuce, fish, and desired toppings. Serve with lime wedges.

Pan-Seared Flounder with Kohlrabi, Carrot, and Apple Slaw

Start to finish: 30 minutes
Serves 4

For the slaw:

3 tablespoons extra-virgin olive oil

1 tablespoon fresh lemon juice

2 teaspoons minced shallot

2 teaspoons fresh thyme leaves

⅛ teaspoon kosher salt

⅛ teaspoon freshly ground black pepper

1 medium kohlrabi, peeled, trimmed, and cut into matchstick-size pieces (2 cups)

1 cup preshredded carrots

1 apple, cored and cut into matchstick-size pieces

For the flounder:

1 tablespoon herbes de Provence

1 teaspoon onion powder

1 teaspoon kosher salt

½ teaspoon freshly ground black pepper

2 tablespoons olive oil, plus more if needed

4 (6-ounce) skinless flounder fillets

1. For the slaw, in a large bowl, whisk together the oil, lemon juice, shallot, thyme, salt, and pepper. Add the kohlrabi, carrots, and apple; toss to combine.

2. For the flounder, in a small bowl, combine the herbes de Provence, onion powder, salt, and pepper.

3. In a large, heavy skillet, heat the oil over medium-high heat. Add the fish and cook for 5 minutes. Turn fillets, adding more oil if necessary. Sprinkle fish with the seasoning, and cook for an additional 5 to 7 minutes or until centers of fillets are just opaque.

5. Serve the fish with the slaw.

Roasted Pork Chops with Olives and Grapes

Prep: 10 minutes

Cook: 20 minutes

Serves 4

1 cup red or purple seedless grapes, some cut in half

⅓ cup small pitted Kalamata olives, some cut in half

1 tablespoon coarsely chopped shallot

4 teaspoons olive oil, divided

¾ teaspoon kosher salt, divided

2 (12- to 14-ounce) bone-in rib or loin pork chops, cut 1¼- to 1½-inch thick (rib-eye or porterhouse pork chops)

½ teaspoon cracked mixed peppercorns

2 teaspoons chopped fresh rosemary leaves

¼ teaspoon dried thyme leaves, crushed

1. Remove the pork chops from the refrigerator 15 minutes before cooking. Preheat the oven to 350°F.

2. In a small bowl, combine the grapes, olives, and shallot. Drizzle with 2 teaspoons of the oil and sprinkle with ¼ teaspoon of the salt. Toss until the grapes and olives are evenly coated.

3. Pat moisture from the chops with paper towels. Rub the remaining 2 teaspoons oil on both sides of the pork chops; season both sides of the chops with the remaining ½ teaspoon salt and the cracked peppercorns.

4. Heat a large cast-iron skillet over medium-high heat. When hot, add the chops and sear on both sides. Arrange the grape mixture around the pork chops in the skillet. Sprinkle the grape mixture and chops with rosemary and thyme. Transfer the skillet to the oven and roast for 15 to 25 minutes or until a thermometer inserted near the center of each chop registers 145°F.

5. Transfer the chops and grape mixture to a serving platter. Cover with foil. Let rest for 3 minutes before serving.

Spiced Beef Burgers with Sweet-and-Sour Red Cabbage

Prep: 25 minutes

Cook: 45 minutes

Serves 4

For the cabbage:

2 tablespoons olive oil

1 cup chopped red onion

6 cups thinly sliced red cabbage

2 Granny Smith apples, peeled, cored, and diced

¾ cup apple juice

3 tablespoons apple cider vinegar

⅛ teaspoon ground cloves

¼ teaspoon ground ginger

⅛ teaspoon ground cinnamon

½ teaspoon freshly ground black pepper

½ teaspoon kosher salt

For the burgers:

1 pound organic grass-fed ground beef

¼ cup finely chopped onion

1 teaspoon lemon zest

¾ teaspoon freshly ground black
pepper

½ teaspoon kosher salt

½ teaspoon ground allspice

1 tablespoon olive oil

½ cup beef-based Basic Bone
Broth (page 252) or purchased
compliant beef bone broth

1. For the cabbage, in a large pot, heat the olive oil over medium-low heat. Add the onion and cook for 6 to 8 minutes or until tender and lightly browned. Add the cabbage and cook for 6 to 8 minutes or until the cabbage is crisp-tender. Add the apples, apple juice, vinegar, cloves, ginger, cinnamon, pepper, and salt. Bring to a boil; reduce the heat to low. Cover and cook for 30 minutes, stirring occasionally. Uncover and cook until the liquid has reduced slightly.

2. Meanwhile, for the burgers, in a large bowl combine the ground beef, onion, lemon zest, pepper, salt, and allspice. Gently mix until everything is well incorporated. Shape the mixture into four ½-inch-thick patties.

3. In a large skillet, heat the oil over medium-high heat. Fry the patties for about 8 minutes or until browned on the exterior and cooked through, turning once. Transfer the burgers to a plate and cover loosely with foil. Add the broth to the skillet, stirring to scrape up the browned bits from the bottom of the skillet. Cook for about 4 minutes or until reduced by half.

4. Drizzle the burgers with the reduced pan juices and serve with the cabbage.

Elimin8 Snacks

Crunchy Veggie Rolls with Homemade Ranch Dressing

Start to finish: 20 minutes

Serves 10

1 (6-ounce) package compliant
sliced turkey or roast beef*

1 small cucumber, peeled and cut
into 10 sticks

½ small jicama, peeled and cut into 10 sticks

1 medium carrot, peeled and cut into 10 sticks

Homemade Ranch Dressing (see below)

1. Place one slice of turkey or beef on a clean work surface. Place one cucumber stick, one jicama stick, and one carrot stick on top of the turkey or beef. Roll up to enclose the vegetables. Serve with dressing. Refrigerate any leftover dressing in an airtight container for up to 1 week.

*NOTE: To make this snack vegan, use Bibb lettuce leaves in place of the sliced turkey or beef.

Homemade Ranch Dressing

In a medium bowl, combine 1 cup Egg-Free Mayonnaise (see page 230), ½ cup canned coconut milk,* ½ teaspoon onion powder, ¼ teaspoon garlic powder, ¼ teaspoon freshly ground black pepper, 1 tablespoon finely chopped fresh dill or 1 teaspoon dried dill, 1 tablespoon finely chopped fresh chives, and 2 teaspoons fresh lemon juice. Whisk to combine.

*NOTE: Coconut milk separates in the can; be sure to empty it into a small bowl and whisk thoroughly before measuring.

Dilled Smoked Salmon–Cucumber Bites

Prep: 15 minutes

Chill: 30 minutes

Serves 8

¼ cup Egg-Free Mayonnaise (page 230)

2 teaspoons chopped fresh dill, plus additional for garnish

¼ teaspoon lemon zest

¼ teaspoon fresh lemon juice

⅛ teaspoon garlic powder

⅛ teaspoon freshly ground white pepper

6 ounces finely chopped compliant hot-smoked salmon*

1 small English cucumber or 8 small Belgian endive leaves

1. In a small bowl, combine the mayonnaise, dill, lemon zest and juice, garlic powder, and white pepper. Stir in the salmon and mix until ingredients are well incorporated. Cover and refrigerate for 30 to 60 minutes to blend flavors.

2. Meanwhile, slice 8 planks from the cucumber at an angle (wrap and refrigerate the remaining cucumber).

3. To serve, spoon the salmon mixture onto the cucumber planks or into the endive leaves. Garnish with fresh dill.

*NOTE: Read the label on your smoked salmon. Some varieties contain sugar and other undesirable ingredients. Hot-smoked salmon that contains only salmon, salt, and woodsmoke is available at most large Whole Foods markets.

Fig and Olive Tapenade

Start to finish: 10 minutes

Serves 6 to 8

⅓ cup chopped dried figs

½ cup pitted Kalamata olives

⅓ cup pitted green olives

1 to 2 tablespoons extra-virgin olive oil

2 teaspoons compliant balsamic vinegar

½ teaspoon minced fresh rosemary

¼ teaspoon minced fresh thyme

1 small garlic clove, chopped

Prosciutto Chips (page 244)

1. Place the figs in a food processor. Cover and process until minced. Add the Kalamata and green olives, 1 tablespoon oil, vinegar,

rosemary, thyme, and garlic. Cover and process until the olives are finely chopped. If necessary, add enough of the remaining 1 tablespoon oil to reach the desired consistency.

2. Serve with Prosciutto Chips.*

*NOTE: Do not season the Prosciutto Chips after baking if they are to be served with this tapenade. To make this dish vegan, serve with vegetables or plantain chips instead.

Lemon-Thyme Parsnip Fries

Prep: 5 minutes
Stand: 10 minutes
Bake: 30 minutes
Serves 4

1 pound small to medium parsnips, peeled	¼ teaspoon freshly ground black pepper
2 tablespoons olive oil or avocado oil	1 tablespoon fresh thyme leaves
½ teaspoon kosher salt	1 teaspoon lemon zest
	Homemade Ranch Dressing (page 241)

1. Preheat the oven to 450°F. Line a large baking sheet with parchment paper.

2. Cut the parsnips into 3×¼-inch julienne (matchsticks). Place the parsnips in a large bowl of ice water; let soak for 10 minutes. Drain the parsnips and pat dry with paper towels. Place the parsnips in a large bowl. Drizzle the oil over the parsnips; toss to coat. Sprinkle with salt and pepper; toss to combine. Arrange the parsnips in an even layer on the prepared baking sheet. Bake the parsnips for 30 minutes or until tender and starting to brown, stirring occasionally.

3. Sprinkle the fries with the fresh thyme leaves and lemon zest. Serve with the ranch dressing for dipping.

Prosciutto Chips, Three Ways

Prep: 5 minutes

Bake: 10 minutes

Serves 4

1 (3- to 4-ounce) package very thinly sliced prosciutto di Parma

Seasoning of choice (see options below)

1. Position a rack in the center of the oven. Preheat the oven to 350°F.

2. Line a large baking pan with parchment paper. Place the prosciutto in a single layer on the prepared baking pan. Bake for 10 to 15 minutes or until starting to crisp; watch carefully to prevent burning. The chips will crisp further as they cool.

3. Transfer the chips to a wire rack with foil, parchment paper, or paper towel underneath. Sprinkle the chips with the seasoning of your choice.

Seasoning 1: Garlic powder and freshly ground black pepper

Seasoning 2: Fresh thyme leaves and lemon zest

Seasoning 3: Herbes de Provence

NOTE: The chips can also be crumbled and sprinkled on top of a soup or salad.

Quick Veggie Pickles

Prep: 25 minutes

Chill: 24 hours

Serves 16 (¼ cup each)

Enough vegetables to fill two (16-ounce) jars with lids, such as sliced beets, carrots, cucumbers, red onion, radishes, and cored and finely sliced fennel bulbs

10 black peppercorns

2 garlic cloves, peeled and crushed

2 (⅛-inch-thick) slices peeled fresh ginger

1 cup apple cider vinegar

1 cup 100% apple juice

1½ teaspoons kosher salt

1. Layer the desired vegetables in two 16-ounce glass jars. Divide the peppercorns, garlic, and ginger between the two jars.

2. In a small saucepan, combine the vinegar, apple juice, and salt. Bring to a boil. Remove from heat and pour the vinegar mixture over the vegetables in jars. Let cool 1 hour. Cover the jars with lids and refrigerate for at least 1 day or up to 3 weeks.

Snack-Size Italian Meatballs

Prep: 20 minutes

Cook: 25 minutes

Serves 16 (2 meatballs each)

¾ pound organic grass-fed ground beef

½ pound organic ground pork

2 tablespoons nutritional yeast

3 tablespoons beef-based Basic Bone Broth (page 252) or purchased compliant bone broth

2 tablespoons coconut flour

2 garlic cloves, minced

1 teaspoon kosher salt

1½ teaspoons Italian seasoning

1 tablespoon minced fresh parsley

Freshly ground black pepper

1. Preheat the oven to 350°F. In a large bowl, combine the beef, pork, nutritional yeast, broth, coconut flour, garlic, salt, Italian seasoning, parsley, and pepper to taste. Using your hands, gently mix until all ingredients are well incorporated.

2. Shape into 32 one-inch meatballs and place on a foil-lined rimmed baking pan.

3. Bake for 25 minutes or until browned on the outside and cooked through.

ELIXIRS AND BROTHS

These medicinal elixirs are perfect for a midmorning break (who needs coffee when these sipping drinks do so much good work for you?), or any time when you need their therapeutic power. There are more here than are listed in the meal plan because I wanted to give you as many therapeutic options as possible. I hope you will try them all, or at least all the ones that address your particular issues.

These elixirs are both Core4 and Elimin8 friendly. Teas and turmeric milk are also excellent for enjoying before bed, for relaxation and calm sleep. Note that many of the ingredients in these recipes may sound unusual and may be hard to find in your regular grocery store. Many of them are also included in the toolboxes in chapter 3. You can find most of these ingredients in well-stocked health food stores, and they should all be available from reputable health food and supplement companies online.

NOTE: If you don't have a juicer, you can make any of the juices in a high-speed blender with just enough filtered water to get a completely liquefied result—the amount may vary, so just add about ¼ cup of water at a time and blend until you get the juice-like result you want.

All of these elixirs take just a few minutes to make and all recipes serve one, but can be doubled to serve two.

Tropical Spice Juice

Made with a base of pineapple, this delicious drink is brimming with goodness perfect for those who suffer from inflammatory issues. Pineapple is full of bromelain, a compound known for its natural enzyme power, which may be helpful for digestion as well as joint pain, allergies, and asthma. Bromelain is excellent at reducing pain and inflammation, and turmeric is also a well-known anti-inflammatory thanks to its rich curcumin content. The dose of cinnamon in this juice helps to add a touch of "spice," while regulating blood sugar levels and reducing your appetite—perfect for those in search of weight-loss juicing recipes.

15 pieces of fresh turmeric root (about 3 inches each—find it in a well-stocked grocery store or health food store)

1 tablespoon cinnamon

2 cucumbers

1 pineapple

Run all the ingredients through a juicer or liquefy in a blender with a little water.

The Green Queen Juice

Sweet and nutritious, this green juice is as wholesome as they come and perfect for those with inflammatory conditions. Kale is a great source of thiamine, protein, folate, riboflavin, magnesium, iron, and phosphorus—but it's also a great source of vitamins A, K, C, and B_6, too. All these vitamins produce great anti-inflammatory effects. At the same time, ginger is a tasty way to relieve pain, and lemons are rich in vitamin C, which is particularly powerful at fighting back against the causes of unnecessary inflammation.

1 bunch of kale

2 kiwifruits

1 lemon wedge

1 slice of ginger

Run all the ingredients through a juicer or liquefy in a blender with some water. If you use a blender, peel the kiwifruits first.

Blueberry Blast Juice

This green blueberry blend could be a great drink to consume before your workouts because it helps to reduce inflammation and gives you a greater boost of energy. When it comes to antioxidants, blueberries are perhaps the most powerful berry around. Their rich anthocyanin content helps to reduce inflammation and offers a range of additional health benefits too.

2 oranges, peeled, seeds removed   2 cups blueberries

2 cups spinach leaves

Run all ingredients through a juicer or liquefy in a blender with water.

Rejuvenating Celery Juice

As simple as this recipe sounds, it is powerful. Celery contains many minerals and nutrients that are great for your gut. I've seen this simple solution do wonders in thousands of patients when consumed consistently. Over time, the juice can help restore your stomach's natural acid, HCL, aiding in healthy digestion and microbiome balance. I recommend drinking up to 16 ounces of fresh celery juice on an empty stomach in the morning. Work up slowly—this juice is quite cleansing, and if you go too fast, you may spend a lot of time in the bathroom.

1 to 2 bunches organic celery

Run the celery through a juicer or liquefy in a blender with water.

Gut-Soothing Ginger and Slippery Elm Tea

Ginger and slippery elm are both anti-inflammatory and healing to your intestinal lining.

1 teaspoon fresh gingerroot   1 teaspoon slippery elm powder

2 cups purified water

Grate the fresh gingerroot into your teapot. Pour 2 cups of water into the pot and boil. Strain. Stir in and dissolve the slippery elm powder.

Refreshing Adrenal-Balancing Iced Tea

These adaptogen plant medicines help calm inflammation and are particularly good at balancing the brain-adrenal (HPA) axis.

1 teaspoon ashwagandha powder

1 teaspoon cinnamon

1 teaspoon holy basil powder

1 teaspoon rhodiola powder

Pour 1 to 2 cups of hot water over the herbs. Let steep for 15 minutes. Pour over ice.

Dr. Will Cole's Gut-Healing Smoothie

This smoothie is therapeutic for your gut. I have a smoothie like this one almost every day.

1 cup full-fat coconut milk

2 tablespoons marine or grass-fed collagen powder

1 tablespoon extra-virgin coconut oil

½ teaspoon probiotic powder

1 teaspoon deglycyrrhizinated licorice (DGL)

1 teaspoon zinc carnosine

1 tablespoon L-glutamine powder

2 cups chopped kale

½ cup frozen organic berries

Combine the ingredients in a blender and blend until smooth.

Adaptogenic Adrenal-Balancing Smoothie

4 Brazil nuts (omit for Elimin8 compliance)

1 cup full-fat coconut milk

1 cup frozen organic berries

1 cup spinach

1 teaspoon ashwagandha powder

1 tablespoon coconut oil or MCT oil

1 tablespoon maca powder

1 teaspoon rhodiola powder

1 scoop collagen peptides

Combine all ingredients in a blender and blend until smooth.

Thyroid-Boosting Smoothie

This smoothie targets your thyroid to improve function and reduce inflammation. If you are using the hormone toolbox, this is a great addition.

1 cup full-fat coconut milk

1 scoop collagen protein

1 tablespoon extra-virgin
  coconut oil

1 cup mixed greens

2 Brazil nuts (omit for Elimin8
  compliance)

1 avocado

1 celery stalk

2 tablespoons dulse flakes

1 tablespoon maca powder

1 cup organic frozen berries

Combine all ingredients in a blender and blend until smooth.

Treg Pumper-Upper Smoothie

Regulatory T cells (Tregs) are your body's inflammation-balancing pow-
erhouses. Support them with this superfood smoothie.

1 cup full-fat coconut milk

3 handfuls greens

Handful frozen berries

1 teaspoon astragalus

1 teaspoon black cumin seed oil

1 teaspoon cat's claw

1 teaspoon raw cacao powder

1 teaspoon curcumin

Combine all ingredients in a blender and blend until smooth.

Sex-Hormone Boosting Elixir

Give your hormones a welcome boost with this elixir, rich with good fats
and medicinal herbs.

1 cup full-fat coconut milk

1 teaspoon cacao powder

1 teaspoon *Mucuna pruriens* powder

1 teaspoon shilajit powder

½ teaspoon cinnamon

Combine all ingredients in a blender and blend well. Pour into a
saucepan and heat for 3 to 5 minutes over medium heat until warm.

Beautifying Blue-Green Mermaid Latte

Not only do the aquatic hues of blue-green algae and spirulina decrease inflammation, but they protect your cells and contain a unique array of antioxidants to help keep your skin and body looking more youthful.

1 cup full-fat coconut milk

1 teaspoon blue-green algae powder or spirulina

½ teaspoon cinnamon

½ teaspoon organic vanilla extract

Place all the ingredients in a saucepan and heat until warm and the ingredients are dissolved. Pour into a mug and enjoy with additional cinnamon sprinkled on top.

Skin-Brightening Lavender Tonic

In the kingdom of adaptogens, pearl is the king of beauty. It's a powerhouse source of aminos that strengthen your hair and nails and nourish your skin. In addition, lavender helps to calm the skin from the inside out.

1½ cups water

1 teaspoon lemon juice

1 teaspoon pearl powder

2 to 3 drops lavender essential oil (be sure to get an edible brand)

Add lemon juice, pearl powder, and lavender essential oil in water and stir until combined.

Anti-Inflammatory Turmeric Milk (Golden Milk)

Turmeric is great for putting out the flames of inflammation. Its benefits are amplified and made more bioavailable when mixed with fats like coconut and spices like black pepper. Ginger is another great anti-inflammatory and gut-healing tool. This drink is great for midmorning, but I also recommend it as an evening drink, especially if you are used to snacking at night.

1 cup coconut milk

1 teaspoon turmeric

½ teaspoon cinnamon

¼ teaspoon ginger powder

Pinch of freshly ground black pepper

Combine all ingredients in a blender and blend well. Pour into a saucepan and heat for 3 to 5 minutes over medium heat until warm.

Basic Bone Broth

Bone broth, the gut super healer, contains many building blocks for your enterocytes, which are the cells lining your gut. The natural blend of gelatin, along with glucosamine, glycine, and minerals, can help calm a reactive, inflamed system. Bone broth can be a therapeutic tool for leaky gut syndrome, diarrhea, constipation, and food sensitivities. If you struggle with histamine intolerance (page 260), I recommend cooking the bones in the broth for a shorter amount of time—closer to 8 hours rather than 48 hours. A pressure cooker will do the work for you even more quickly, with minimum histamine buildup. I make this often and always keep some in my freezer for making soup.

Typically makes about 4 quarts, depending on how much water you add

Choose one for your bones:

1 whole organic chicken or chicken carcass/bones

1 small whole organic turkey, turkey breast, or turkey carcass/ bones

3 to 5 pounds grass-fed beef bones

1 pound fish bones, shrimp shells, or other crustacean shells (mussels, clams, crabs, etc.)

For the broth:

6 garlic cloves

1 onion

2 large carrots, scrubbed and
chopped

3 to 4 organic celery stalks,
chopped

1-inch gingerroot, peeled and
sliced into coins

¼ cup apple cider vinegar

1 teaspoon turmeric powder or
a 3-inch piece of turmeric
root

1 tablespoon chopped fresh
parsley

1 teaspoon Himalayan salt

1. Rinse the bones and place them in the large soup pot or Dutch oven,
   slow cooker, or pressure cooker. Fill the pot three-quarters full of
   water (or up to the maximum fill line) and add the herbs and
   vegetables. Follow these instructions, according to your cooking
   method:

2. **For the stove,** cook over medium-high heat until bubbling, then
   reduce the heat to low and allow to simmer, covered, for at least 8
   hours, adding more water as needed to keep the bones mostly
   covered.

   For the slow cooker, set on low and cover. Cook for at least 8 but no
   more than 10 hours.

   For the pressure cooker, follow the manufacturer's instructions for
   broth or soup.

3. After cooking, allow the broth to cool, then pour it through a
   fine-mesh strainer into a large bowl, discarding the solids. Transfer
   to mason jars to store in the fridge, or freezer-safe containers for
   longer-term storage.

Galangal Broth

Not to be confused with ginger, galangal is its own root but still part of
the same rhizome family of plants, which makes its appearance to

ginger very similar. But while they may look the same, each has its own unique taste and texture. Unlike regular ginger, galangal can only be sliced, not grated, due to its harder exterior. Galangal also has a much stronger flavor than the spicy taste of ginger—galangal packs a punch to the taste buds with its sharp, extra citrusy, piney flavor. Galangal is also referred to as Thai ginger due to its popularity in Thai, Malaysian, and Indonesian cuisines and has been used for centuries in Ayurvedic medicine and remedies in other Asian cultures. What the galangal root lacks in collagen and other nutrients found only in bone broth it makes up for with its other powerful compounds that work to heal the gut through various means. Without a doubt, galangal broth is one of my top ways to improve gut health. Fresh galangal can be found at health food markets like Whole Foods, and it is also sold online. If you can't find fresh galangal, you can also buy the dried, ground variety. Generally, for every tablespoon of fresh galangal use a quarter-teaspoon of dried, ground galangal.

Makes 3 quarts

12 cups vegetable broth

1-inch piece galangal, sliced into rounds

3 stalks lemongrass

3 green onions, sliced

3 stalks celery, including greens

4 kaffir lime leaves

½ teaspoon sea salt

1 teaspoon freshly ground black pepper

3–4 cilantro sprigs, for garnish

1. Heat the vegetable stock in a large soup pot over medium to high heat and bring to a boil.

2. Add the galangal, lemongrass, green onions, celery, and kaffir lime leaves.

3. Let boil for 10 minutes.

4. Remove from the heat and let stand for 20 minutes to allow the broth to absorb the nutrients and flavors.

5. Strain the broth, discarding the solids, and season with salt and pepper.

6. Garnish with fresh cilantro and serve hot.

NOTE: Once cooled, this broth can be stored in mason jars and frozen for later use.

7

REINTEGR8: TESTING YOUR OLD FAVORITES

Now that you have learned what it is like to live without those foods you thought you loved, it's time to test whether your body loves them, too—or whether the preferences you had before you started the elimination phase are at odds with your biology. You will be working through a systematic reintroduction of the foods you hope to bring back into your life, but this is much more than a testing period. This is a time of self-reflection. Don't assume you will still want everything you used to eat, or even that any of those foods will taste the same or evoke the same response from your body that they did before. Think deeply about the foods that were once a part of your daily or weekly life. Do you miss them or do you feel better without them?

It is common, after the elimination phase, to experience a change in preferences. Whereas once you might have craved candy, potato chips, or a Starbucks Caramel Frappuccino, you may notice that now those things don't sound as appealing. They may even sound unappealing. You have been through an intense palate cleansing and whole-body deep cleaning, so as you reintroduce foods, you may well find that the things you used to eat, maybe even without thinking, now taste strange, too sweet, too greasy, or too artificial when you reintroduce them. Trust your current reaction more than your previous inclination, because your body is at its most centered and discerning after the elimination phase. The way food tastes to you right now is how the food *actually tastes*, now that your body has reduced its inflammation and your senses are more in tune. This is the time to test your true reactions.

But don't let your newly minted awareness end at the first bite. Notice a ripple effect throughout your body with every new tested food. How does the food taste as you continue to chew it or take more bites? What sensations do you notice immediately after you eat it? How do you feel fifteen minutes later? An hour later? A day later? This is what we will explore in this chapter.

One by one and step by step, we will introduce some of the foods you have eliminated—the ones you still think you want to bring back into your life—and you will evaluate your body's responses as you go. I'll walk you through exactly how to do it so you know when you are reacting to something and when you aren't. If you find that some things are not reactive for you and you want to eat them again, I'll show you how to work them back into your life in new and fresh ways.

WHAT DO YOU WANT TO BRING BACK?

Most of my patients have at least some foods they want to try to reintegrate—but as you assess what you can and can't live without, think about how you feel now and how you felt before. Weigh that awareness against your feelings about certain foods. Maybe you can do without gluten, but you have your fingers crossed for gluten-free grains like brown rice and corn. Maybe you feel great without sugar but would love to be able to eat nut butter, black beans, or scrambled eggs again. Maybe you want to know that if you genuinely crave some goat cheese, fresh tomatoes, a baked potato, lentil soup, or a handful of almonds, you can indulge your craving without making yourself ill or suffering from a recurrence of your past symptoms. All those foods can be great, nutrient-dense options that can benefit your health . . . *if* your body loves them, too.

Or you may not want to bring *anything* back at this point, if you are feeling relief from your old symptoms. To some people, eight weeks (or even four weeks) seem like an eternity without coffee, cheese, chocolate, or whatever, but to others, eight weeks fly by, and when I tell them it is time to start reintroducing, they look at me with panic. They aren't ready yet.

If you feel like your body has been a little slower to react, or if you switched to Elimin8 from the Core4 halfway through and you are still making progress, or if you don't feel mentally ready to leave this place of healing and ultra-clean eating, then go longer. That's completely fine! You do not need to live in fear of foods, but the foods you have been eating on this program are nourishing your body, taking you closer to your health goals, and teaching you more about what does and does not work for you. This is a good thing, and one I want you to continue to explore if you feel it's right for you to do so. Don't reintegrate any food until you feel ready and are certain that you want it back in your life. There is no reason not to continue with the elimination phase of this program for as long as you feel you need it. You could go twelve, sixteen, even twenty-plus weeks before reintegrating anything, if you are feeling great and want to keep it up. In fact, you could stay in the elimination phase forever, if you wanted to. It is nutritionally dense and complete, which is exactly what your body needs in the long term. If you do choose to stay with your Core4 or Elimin8 plan longer, just be sure to stay focused on getting lots of different vegetables, healthy fats, and clean protein. Reintroduction is only for those people who want to bring back some of their eliminated foods. It's optional for any foods you are fine living without.

However, as I said, it's also okay to want to try to bring back foods you miss and genuinely hope to eat going forward. I want to help you find the best way possible to do that with proper reintroduction.

IF YOU ARE STILL HAVING SOME SYMPTOMS

Every so often, someone goes through the elimination phase of this program and still has some lingering symptoms. Don't be discouraged by this. You may just need some fine-tuning and optimizing of your plan. Wellness is a journey. If this sounds like you, then you may need to continue the elimination phase a little bit longer or you may have slightly less common sensitivities that we haven't yet pinpointed. Not sure? Pull out that list of the eight most bothersome symptoms that you made at the beginning after the quiz (page 54). Do you still have some of these? If so, it's possible that you have a sensitivity to:

1. Histamines

2. Salicylates

3. FODMAPs

4. Oxalates

After your elimination phase, if your persistent symptoms relate to digestion issues, skin problems, mood swings, neurological symptoms, congestion issues, or any sign of inflammation, they could also be a sign of these sensitivities. (If they are none of these, check out the information at the end of this section about getting individualized care.) Let's take a closer look at these.

Histamines

Histamines (and other amines) are compounds produced by your immune system that trigger a defense against allergens (and also work as neurotransmitters). When they get released inappropriately or in excess, they can cause many kinds of symptoms in those who are sensitive to them—from allergy symptoms like an itchy throat and a stuffy nose to skin symptoms, digestive problems, joint pain, and neurological symptoms. If you notice any of these symptoms after eating cured meat or fermented foods like kombucha, wine, or sauerkraut, this may be a sign that you are histamine sensitive.[1] In this case, try eliminating all histamine-rich foods for another two weeks before you begin the reintroduction phase and see if that makes a difference. If it does, then reduce or eliminate these foods until you see the changes in your health that you are looking for. This may mean permanent or long-term removal of these foods, depending on your healing journey and what that looks like for your body. Gut issues like SIBO (small intestinal bacterial overgrowth) can be the culprit for histamine intolerance (and FODMAP intolerance; see below). Addressing SIBO is a step for some people with histamine or FODMAP intolerance.

HIGH-HISTAMINE FOODS

Here are the foods with the highest content of histamine, foods that could cause an overload:

- Alcohol (especially beer and wine)

- Bone broth

- Canned food

- Cheese, especially aged cheese

- Chocolate

- Eggplant

- Fermented foods (kefir, kimchi, yogurt, sauerkraut)

- Legumes (especially fermented soybeans, chickpeas, and peanuts)

- Mushrooms

- Nuts, especially cashews and walnuts

- Processed foods

- Shellfish

- Smoked meat products (bacon, salami, salmon, ham)

- Spinach

- Vinegar

FOODS THAT RELEASE HISTAMINE

These foods are low in histamines but can trigger the release of histamine, thus creating problems for people with histamine intolerance:

- Avocados

- Bananas

- Citrus fruits (lemons, limes, oranges, grapefruit)

- Strawberries

- Tomatoes

DIAMINE OXIDASE (DAO) ENZYME BLOCKERS

These foods block the enzyme that controls histamine, which can cause higher levels in some people:

- Alcohol

- Energy drinks

- Teas (black, green, yerba maté)

Salicylates

Salicylates are compounds found in pain medications like aspirin as well as in beauty and skin products, but in the context of food, salicylates are naturally found in many plant foods. In certain plant foods, salicylates act as a defense mechanism to protect the plant. The symptoms of salicylate intolerance[2] can be similar to those of histamine intolerance: neurological, digestive, or skin reactions. If you think you might have this intolerance, try eliminating these salicylate-rich foods and see if it helps:

- Almonds

- Apricots

- Avocados

- Blackberries

- Cherries

- Coconut oil

- Dates

- Dried fruits

- Endive

- Gherkins

- Grapes

- Green olives

- Guavas

- Honey

- Nightshades (peppers, eggplant, tomatoes, potatoes)

- Olive oil

- Oranges

- Pineapple

- Plums/prunes

- Tangelos

- Tangerines

- Water chestnuts

FODMAPs

If you notice gastrointestinal symptoms when you eat high-fructose fruit and certain vegetables, legumes, sweeteners, and grains—especially wheat—then your problem may be a sensitivity to fermentable oligosaccharides, disaccharides, monosaccharides, and polyols, or FODMAPs for short. These are a group of carbohydrates that can cause IBS-type symptoms (like constipation, diarrhea, stomach cramping, and bloating) in some people.[3] If this sounds like you, try eliminating the most potent sources of FOD-MAPs for two weeks and see if that helps. If it does, consider going low FODMAP by reducing or eliminating most of these foods and then reintroducing them slowly and one at a time (using the reintroduction techniques in this chapter). You may be tolerant of some FODMAPs but not of others, so it's good to test these one at a time (or in small groups, since the list is long) to see if your symptoms improve:

- Artichoke

- Asparagus

- Bananas

- Beets

- Cabbage

- Cashews

- Carob powder

- Cauliflower

- Coconut water

- Dairy products, all types from cow's milk: cheese, milk, cream, ice cream, sour cream, yogurt

- Fruit juice of any kind

- Garlic

- Gluten—all products that contain wheat, barley, rye, or spelt

- Green beans

- High-fructose fruits (all except berries, limes, lemons, and melons)

- Honey

- Legumes

- Mushrooms

- Onions, all types (including shallots and scallions)

- Peas

- Sauerkraut

- Soy

- Sugar alcohols (often used in sugar-free sweet products, these include inulin, isomalt, maltitol, mannitol, sorbitol, xylitol)

Oxalates

Oxalates are plant compounds that can bind to minerals to form calcium oxalate and iron oxalate. This can happen in the digestive tract, kidneys, or urinary tract. In oxalate-sensitive people, this can drive inflammation in these areas.[4]

Foods higher in oxalates include:

- Beets

- Cocoa

- Kale

- Peanuts

- Spinach

- Sweet potatoes

- Swiss chard

Cooking vegetables can lower their oxalate content.

WHEN TO CONSULT A FUNCTIONAL MEDICINE PRACTITIONER

If none of these elimination efforts solves your problem and you are still struggling, if you aren't seeing the level of change you want to see, or if you have a serious health issue, then you may need more personalized intervention than I can provide in a book. I suggest consulting a qualified functional medicine practitioner who can sit down with you, evaluate your symptoms, ask you questions, and work with you in person to get to the root of your issues. We consult with people around the world via webcam consultation (www.drwillcole.com), or to find a functional medicine doc near you, go to functionalmedicine.org.

CREATING YOUR REINTEGR8 PLAN

It's test time! Did you study? Just kidding—you've been "studying" for this test for the last four or eight weeks, and now it's time to find out the score. You've eliminated four or eight food items, and now you are going to test them, one at a time, in a very specific order—from least potentially inflammatory and problematic to most potentially inflammatory—monitoring your reactions to each one.

Each test takes three days. Remember, this is no time to be in a hurry. You are experimenting, and this is the best way to keep the experiment accurate. Foods need to come back in one at a time. If you start eating everything you want all at once—a pepperoni pizza, for example—and you have a terrible stomachache or headache or joint pain afterward, you won't know whether it was from the grains or the eggs in the crust, the dairy cheese, or the tomato sauce. You must isolate these inflammatory triggers one at a time, and then maybe you will discover that you *can* have pizza, as long as the crust is gluten-free, or the cheese is non-dairy, or you have white sauce instead of red sauce. This is a process not meant to be frustratingly slow, but an accurate reflection of your body's reactions. Be patient with your body and yourself during this time and you will reap the rewards of all your hard work. As you work through your tests, continue to adhere to all other aspects of your track. Remember that you are bringing in only *one* previously eliminated food at a time.

Because reactions can take a few days to show up, this is the necessary timeline for you to get the most accurate information. You might not react immediately to a food, but then you might get terrible reflux the next morning or a splitting headache on the second day or a cascade of other reactions over the next few days. Thankfully, though, because of your diligence over the previous weeks, you're much more prepared to handle these, so be introspective and observant. You are about to engage in a long, relaxed, extended conversation with your body about your mutual future. "Hey, body. I was thinking lentil soup. Let's try some lentils and see how we like them, and we can discuss. Then maybe we can talk about goat cheese." With every reintroduced food, you will carefully track any reactions. Everyone reacts differently to food, so this is the best way for you to see and know how your body feels after introducing each one.

HOW WILL YOU KNOW IF YOU ARE REACTING?

When your inflammation is high and you have symptoms all the time, it can be difficult to assess when or whether you are reacting to any particular food or influence. Now it will be easier. Your system is centered, clean, and calm, and you are likely to get a more dramatic reaction from certain foods than you did before you started the elimination phase. When you do get a reaction, consider that to be a protest from your body—a message that it does not like that food. Now that you are listening, take that body wisdom to heart. There are many delicious foods, and if your body reacts badly to some of them, you will be happier and healthier if you leave those foods behind.

Reactions can come in many forms. As you begin to test foods, any of the following symptoms count as a reaction and you should record them, even if you aren't 100 percent sure they came from the food you ate:

- Any aggravation or recurrence of your past symptoms that went away during the last four or eight weeks

- Headaches or migraines

- Any digestive symptoms (bloating, nausea, constipation, diarrhea, heartburn, abdominal pain)

- Any skin problems (itching, rashes, hives, acne breakouts, sudden appearance of dry flaky skin)

- Eyes or mouth itching, irritated, or burning, especially right after eating a food

- Sudden nasal congestion, itching, or dripping, especially right after eating a food

- Increased heart rate: racing heart, palpitations, skipped heartbeats

- Joint pain, joint stiffness, especially on both sides of the body at the same time or all over

- All-over muscle aches or stiff muscles

- Feeling feverish

- Brain fog symptoms, such as trouble concentrating, focusing, or remembering things, especially if this has abated in the last eight weeks and suddenly comes back or gets noticeably worse

- Sudden fatigue

- Sudden mood changes—depression, anxiety, panic, nervousness, sense of doom

- Retaining water—limbs and face look thicker, rings don't fit, clothes leave marks in your skin

- Sudden weight gain of a pound or two

- Sleep inconsistency or inability to fall or stay asleep

Remember that your body should have the final word, and if you do react to any of the foods you test, I hope you will stay willing to give up that food potentially for good—or at least for another eight weeks, at which point you could test again. You may just need more time to heal.

If you test a food and feel great with no symptoms, don't be afraid to reintegrate that food. Your body has told you that it doesn't have a problem with it.

Now it's time to make some decisions. Think about what you want to have back in your life and what you can do without. Put a check mark next to every item you would like to test for reintegration, keeping an open mind that any of the foods you check could potentially be reactive and your reintegration test may not yield the all clear you're hoping for. It's okay to check only one, and it's okay to check them all.

Core4

☐ **Grains.** Many react, but not everyone. Do you want to try bringing grains back so that you can have bread, flour tortillas, bagels, crackers, and all those old standards? If so, you will be bringing in gluten-free grains first (like rice, corn, quinoa) and end with gluten-containing grains, especially wheat. As you do this, listen closely to your body. Don't dismiss symptom recurrence just because you think you really need bread.

☐ **Dairy.** If you aren't as satisfied with the plant-based versions and you want to be able to put cream in your coffee again or have real cheese or ice cream, check the dairy box. You'll start by testing butter and cream, and work up from there. You may also find you can tolerate dairy products made with goat's or sheep's milk, but not cow's milk, or that you can tolerate only dairy products with A2 casein. (For more about this, see page 92).

☐ **Added sweeteners.** I recommend avoiding these except for special occasions, but you may need to avoid them all the time. If you would like to try bringing them back, you will start by testing natural sweeteners first, like pure maple syrup, raw honey, and coconut or date sugar. These may agree with you, and white sugar may not. If you do okay with these, you can choose to test white sugar, but even if you don't react to it, please limit your consumption. Over time, too much refined sugar is almost guaranteed to ramp up your inflammation again, no matter who you are. I do not recommend bringing back any food containing high-fructose corn syrup or any artificial sweetener—don't even bother testing these. Consider them on your permanently prohibited list. They are no good for anyone.

☐ **Inflammatory oils.** As with sugar, I recommend using these sparingly, even if you don't react to them. If you don't want to worry that you are getting some industrial seed oil in a restaurant meal or a packaged food occasionally, then see how you react to things like canola oil, corn oil, soybean oil, and vegetable oil. A low level of usage may be okay for you.

Elimin8

If you did the Elimin8 track, you can try reintegrating any of the four foods on the Core4 list previously mentioned, as well as any of the four following foods. Many of these foods are quite healthful and just fine to eat often *if you don't react*. If you do, then consider these to be examples of foods that are potentially healthful for some people but just don't work for you personally.

☐ **Nuts and seeds.** Delicious as snack foods and as additions to many dishes from entrées to desserts, nuts and seeds have valuable nutrition, but some people can find them difficult to digest. If you want to try introducing them, check this box. You will be testing one variety at a time, starting with soaked versions, which are always a healthier and more digestible choice for everyone. You will move on to raw, then roasted, if you want to be able to enjoy those on occasion. You may discover that some nuts and seeds work for you and others don't. For example, many people can eat almonds or walnuts without a problem but have reactions to cashews or pistachios. You may also find that you do fine with a certain amount, but if you eat too many of them they cause you some symptoms.

☐ **Egg whites or whole eggs.** If you check this box, you'll reintroduce yolks first, and if those are fine, you can try the whole egg. Many people do fine with eggs, but not everyone does, so if you love eggs for breakfast, find out your status. You may find that you can eat egg yolks with no problem, but egg whites cause you more inflammation issues. Duck eggs are generally better tolerated over chicken eggs.

☐ **Nightshades.** Most problematic for those who suffer from a lot of joint and skin inflammation as well as digestive issues, nightshades are normally fine for others, and a good source of antioxidants. If you miss salsa or pepper steak or eggplant on your pizza, check this box.

☐ **Legumes.** If you can tolerate them, legumes can be a good source of protein and fiber. Some people aren't fans of legumes, but if you love them and would prefer to get more of your protein from them, check this box. When you reintegrate legumes, you will try lentils and mung beans first, as they are typically more easily tolerated than other legumes. Next try other legumes you like, such as black beans, pinto beans, or white beans. Try soy last, if you really want to be able to enjoy it going forward. If you are tolerant of soy, you may also be able to tolerate edamame, soy milk, and tofu, but always choose non-GMO, preferably organic products. No matter your reaction, I suggest continuing to avoid processed soy products like "veggie dogs" and "veggie burgers" that are not freshly made.

These are the foods I most want to reintroduce (you can have fewer than eight):

1. _____

2. _____

3. _____

4. _____

5. _____

6. _____

7. _____

8. _____

Tracking Your Reaction

Each test takes three days, and you will introduce each food like this:

- Record your test food on your reintroduction test worksheet (see page 280).

- Try one bite of the test food. The food should not include anything else or be part of a complex dish. For example, try tomato sauce alone, not tomato sauce on spaghetti or pizza crust.

- Wait 15 minutes. See if you have any physical reaction, like those listed on pages 267–68. If you do, record it.

- After the 15 minutes have passed, have ¼ cup of the food (if appropriate) or three bites.

- Wait 15 more minutes. Record any additional reaction or worsening of your initial reaction. If you are feeling bad at this point, stop. Assume your body does not like that food right now. Take it back out of your diet for at least thirty more days, then retest it.

- If you still feel fine, have ½ cup more of that food, or six bites, and wait 2 hours. Pay close attention to how you feel during those 2 hours and record any symptoms. If you get symptoms, stop. Assume you are reacting to that food. Take it out of your diet for thirty days and then retest—or take it out forever, if you'd like. You may need to reduce your inflammation further before your body can handle it.

- If all is clear after 2 hours, have a full portion (the amount you would normally eat) of the food, then wait for three days. Do not eat that food again for three days. Throughout those three days, record any reactions. *Do not test any other food.* Your diet should remain the same as it was during your four- or eight-week elimination phase. You are isolating that one food, so don't confuse the test with additional food introductions or the cause of any symptoms won't be clear.

■ If after three days you still have no reaction, your test was successful. Bring that food back into your diet. If you had symptoms during the three days, that food is suspect. Remove it again for at least thirty days, at which point you could retest it if you want to try again. Your body is telling you that it doesn't like that food, so it may be best to say goodbye to it and focus on all the other foods that make you feel awesome.

■ Start the next test with the next food.

NOTE: Quantities listed here don't apply to chia seeds, flaxseed, butter, or spices. Use the same process for these foods but introduce them in smaller amounts and gradually increase to the amount you would normally eat during any given meal.

Remember that this process is about seeing how your body responds to the reintegration of this food item. It can be easy to get carried away when you first taste something you have missed, so stick to the reintroduction portions as I've specified.

Order of Reintegration

You will test the generally mildest, least reactive foods first, and the foods that are most commonly reactive in most people last. If you did the Elimin8 track, start with number 1. Core4 folks, start with number 5. It is very important to go in this order. If you do not want to reintegrate these, move on to the next one.

1. Nuts and seeds (in order of least likely to be inflammatory to most likely to be inflammatory).

■ Unsweetened seed milks, like hemp milk

■ Seed butters, like unsweetened sunflower butter and tahini

■ Soaked flaxseed and/or chia seeds added to a smoothie (they get gelatinous when soaked, so best to add them to something—otherwise, the texture may be unappealing)

- Other seeds, soaked for at least 8 hours or overnight, rinsed, and dried in a dehydrator or an oven set at a low temperature until crunchy again. Then test.

- Unsoaked raw seeds (although ideally, I think all seeds should be soaked to break down lectins and make their nutrients more bioavailable—but this test will help you to know if you can handle them this way on occasion)

- Unsoaked roasted seeds, like sunflower, pumpkin, and sesame seeds. Eat these sparingly, even if you don't react.

- Unsweetened nut milks without additives, such as almond milk and hazelnut milk. These are easiest to digest. Do not try cashew milk yet.

- Smooth (not chunky) nut butters. These are also easier to digest—try almond butter and walnut butter. Do not try cashew butter yet.

- Whole raw nuts. Soak for at least 8 hours, rinse, dry, place them in a dehydrator or an oven set at a low temperature until crispy again, then test.

- Unsoaked raw nuts—although ideally all nuts, like seeds, should be soaked.

- Unsoaked roasted nuts, such as almonds, walnuts, pecans, hazelnuts, and macadamia nuts. As with roasted seeds, eat these sparingly, even if you don't react. They are the most inflammatory form of nuts.

- Test pistachios and cashews last, as they tend to be the most inflammatory of all the nuts.

2. Eggs. When testing eggs, test the yolks only first. Three days later, you can test the whole egg. Ducks eggs tend to be better tolerated than chicken eggs.

3. Nightshades. Introduce these in the following order (testing only the ones you are sure you want to reintroduce):

- Bell peppers (or any sweet peppers)

- White, purple, red, or yellow potatoes, peeled

- White, purple, red, or yellow potatoes, including the skin

- Eggplants

- Tomatoes, raw

- Tomato sauce

- Nightshade spices like cayenne pepper and paprika (introduce one at a time)

- Chili peppers (or any spicy peppers)

4. Legumes. Try them one at a time, in this order:

- Lentils and/or mung beans. These should be soaked for at least 8 hours and rinsed before cooking or cooked in a pressure cooker to break down lectins. For convenience, certain canned brands use a pressure cooker.

- Any other bean (like black, pinto, white, adzuki, etc.), soaked for at least 8 hours and rinsed before cooking or cooked in a pressure cooker to break down lectins

- Organic canned beans, rinsed before heating

- Organic peanuts, including roasted and peanut butter without additives. Valencia peanuts tend to be the most easily tolerated.

Now try soy, in this order (note that I do not ever recommend non-organic, GMO soy food of any type):

- Edamame

- Fermented organic non-GMO soy products: tempeh, miso, natto, tamari (not regular soy sauce, which contains gluten)

- Non-fermented, minimally processed organic non-GMO soy products: fresh tofu, fresh soy milk

- Organic prepared products containing soy but with no other ingredients you haven't already been eating, such as high-quality whole-food veggie burgers. (Do not eat products containing soy isolate.)

Coffee and Black Tea

At this time you can try reintroducing coffee and/or black tea if you enjoy these drinks. We all have different tolerances to caffeinated drinks. If you notice you feel jittery or anxious or get digestive symptoms from drinking coffee or black tea (especially coffee), then decrease the amount you are drinking. Some people don't do well on any amount of coffee and do better on green, white, or herbal teas instead. You can test this for yourself now to see what your body loves.

5. Dairy. Many people react differently to different types of dairy, so if you want to bring this back in, reintroduce dairy products in the following order (note that I do not recommend ever reintroducing nonorganic conventional cow's milk):

- Grass-fed butter

- Grass-fed cream

- Fermented grass-fed kefir and/or yogurt made from goat's or sheep's milk

- Fermented grass-fed kefir and/or yogurt made from the milk of cows that produce primarily A2 casein (page 92)

- Fermented grass-fed kefir and/or yogurt made from the milk of cows that produce primarily A1 casein

- Goat's or sheep's cheese

- Goat's or sheep's milk and/or cream

- Organic raw cheese made from cow's milk (like raw mozzarella)

- Organic regular cheese (like cheddar, Gouda, Muenster, etc.) made from cow's milk

- Organic regular cow's milk, full fat

- Organic regular cow's milk, reduced fat

6. Added sweetener. Although the natural types contain some micronutrients and tend to be less disruptive to blood sugar, too much of any sweetener is not a great idea. If you do need a little more sweetness in your life, however, test sweeteners in this order:

- Start with natural sweeteners: stevia, monk fruit, and sugar alcohols like xylitol, maple syrup, honey, date sugar, coconut sugar, and agave syrup. Test the ones you think you are most likely to use. If you know you won't use it, don't bother testing it. You certainly do not need any added sweetener in your diet. Be sure to test each one of these separately, and note that many people have gastrointestinal reactions to sugar alcohols, so pay close attention to your reactions to these, if you want to reintroduce them.

- Test white cane sugar last.

- I do not ever recommend consuming high-fructose corn syrup or any artificial sweeteners. These high-fructose, highly refined products are too hard on the liver.

7. Inflammatory oils. I do not recommend having these often, even if you don't obviously react to them. Test the types you are most likely to want to use, such as canola oil or corn oil. If you don't plan to use it, don't bother testing it. You certainly don't need any of these in your diet.

8. Grains. Start with **gluten-free grains,** including rice, corn, and quinoa, in this order:

- White rice, soaked and drained before cooking

- Brown rice, soaked and drained before cooking

- Fresh corn

- Gluten-free oats made into oatmeal, without any additives you haven't been eating already

- Whole grains (like gluten-free oats, quinoa, millet, or amaranth), soaked and drained before cooking

- Prepared corn products, like corn tortillas, corn chips (not fried in inflammatory oils), and polenta (without additives)

- Baked goods made with gluten-free flour (without any added ingredients you haven't already been eating, and without added sweetener), such as gluten-free bread or tortillas made with brown rice flour

Next, try **gluten-containing grains and flours** (wheat, rye, barley, spelt, etc.). Try them one at a time, because you may react to some but not others. Here is your order:

- Fermented breads, like whole-grain sourdough with minimal ingredients

- Organic minimally processed whole grains, like barley in soup, bulgur wheat in tabbouleh salad, or simple spelt or rye bread

- Refined versions, like French baguette or white sourdough

- Conventional bread, snack foods like pretzels and crackers, bagels, English muffins, and baked goods without added ingredients you aren't already eating. I don't ever recommend conventional snack foods that contain added inflammatory oils or hydrogenated fats

Reintegrating Alcohol

We all know that alcohol, especially in excess, isn't good for you, but for some people, small amounts (like an occasional glass of wine) can have health benefits. If you *needed* that glass of wine every day after work, you have likely broken that bad habit by now, but what if you want to bring it back in, in moderation? Find out if this will work for you in eight short days, following my process for reintegrating the occasional alcoholic drink. When you are not testing any other food, enjoy 1 glass of your desired drink. This drink should not exceed these amounts:

- 6 ounces red or white wine

- 12 ounces beer (most beer contains gluten, so if you know you cannot have gluten, don't drink beer unless it is gluten-free)

- 1 ounce spirits (vodka, rum, whiskey, tequila, etc.)

- 2 ounces liqueur (liqueurs may contain sugar, so if you know you cannot have inflammatory sweeteners, don't drink liqueur made with those, and avoid any mixer containing high-fructose corn syrup)

If you notice any reaction while you are drinking, stop immediately. If no reaction occurs, wait seven more days. If you don't have any reaction within that time frame, reintroduce alcohol back into your diet permanently, but please do practice moderation. Too much of any of these will be inflammatory.

REINTRODUCTION TEST WORKSHEET

Here is a sample worksheet for you to copy as many times as you need for the foods that you want to reintroduce.

TEST FOOD	
TEST	**REACTION**
1 bite	
After 15 minutes: 3 bites or ¼ cup	
15 minutes after that: 6 bites or ½ cup	
2 hours later: full portion	
Full portion: Day One *Do not have this food again for the next three days—we* *are tracking your reaction to a single serving.*	
Day Two	
Day Three	
Reintroduce? Y/N	
Notes	

The truth at last! Congratulations on successfully completing the Reinteg8 part of this program. Now you know what foods work for you and what foods don't. You know what foods your body loves and what foods your body simply doesn't like. This is the basis of your new way of life going forward—a life full of delicious foods you love that love you back, and no more of the foods that plague you, inflame you, and make you feel like less than your spectacular self. In the next chapter, I'll help you integrate all this information back into your life. Because this is living—diet-free, dogma-free, and just all around free.

If you want to test more foods in addition to your initial top eight, such as foods high in histamines, salicylates, FODMAPs, oxalates (pages 260–65), or any new food you suspect you might be reacting to, go forward using this same technique. This is a tool to use for the rest of your life, if you should ever need it again, because sometimes, food sensitivities develop when they were not present before. This is the best way to stick with the foods that fuel your health, rather than compromise it.

Now for the record:

Foods I have successfully reintroduced without symptoms—my body loves them!

_____

_____

_____

_____

_____

_____

_____

_____

Foods that still cause symptoms—my body doesn't like these.

_____

_____

_____

_____

_____

_____

_____

_____

8

CRE8: HOW TO DESIGN YOUR NEW, PERSONALIZED FOOD AND LIFE PLAN

You are unique, and now you have the proof. You have a list of foods that are good for you but not necessarily for anyone else. You have a list of foods you don't tolerate, whether anyone else does or not. This is personal knowledge that applies only to you. These lists also comprise the building blocks you can use to create a dietary environment for yourself that nourishes you and builds your health. No longer will you unknowingly eat in a way that feeds inflammation. You have the knowledge to make the choice to eat the foods your body loves and thrives on.

After four or eight days of stepping into an anti-inflammatory lifestyle and four or eight weeks of living it, you may also have discovered that you are more disciplined than you knew. Now that it's over, it's time to consider what aspects of the program you want to continue with, and that discipline may be one thing you will need to call on as you move ahead.

MAKE YOUR PERSONAL LIFE PLAN

The first thing I advise my patients to do after the successful completion of an elimination diet is to create a personalized life plan. This is your list of safe foods that you know your body loves. You can carry it with you wherever you go or put it somewhere you will see it often—in your smartphone, on a piece of paper you keep in your wallet, or attached to your refrigerator. After a while, you will have it memorized. Start with the list you made at the end of the last chapter, of reintegrated foods that work for you. Add all the good foods you enjoyed during the four- or eight-week inflammation-cooling phase. Browse the food list (starting on page 108) to find other good possibilities. This is your personal life plan. Whenever you need to find something to eat, consult this list to keep feeding your health. You can always add to this list as you discover more foods (like awesome new vegetables, fruits, kinds of fish, etc.). When in doubt, you can always test new foods by subjecting them to the same elimination diet process.

I also advise making a list of foods that you have chosen to avoid, to keep your inflammation in check. You might write it on the back of your life plan. Start with the foods you listed at the end of the last chapter that did not work for you. Add any other foods that cause a reaction in you, such as any you might have discovered testing for histamines, FODMAPs, salicylates, or oxalates (pages 260–65). You can also add any foods you choose not to eat for any other reason. For example, you may not react to added sweeteners, but you may choose to avoid them anyway.

These lists can be a touchstone for you as you move through your life enjoying food *normally* without the unnatural adherence to a strict diet plan or subservience to diet dogma. You are stepping into your new life now, and the truth is that you can eat anything you want to eat—but you are also armed with knowledge about your own body, so your decisions are now informed.

This is how real-life eating works. Your "plan" is simple. You have a list of foods that you know build your health. Eat more of those. You also have a list of foods you know are inflammatory for you. Choose whether or not you want to eat those, knowing the consequences. You are in charge! Rather than feeling limited, consider that you have endless possibilities ahead of you.

CREATE A WEEK OF DEFAULT MEALS

The next thing I help my patients do is to brainstorm a default week of meals to fall back on whenever they can't think of what to eat or when they don't have time to plan something complicated. Base your week of default meals on your personal life plan. Use one of the blank meal plan forms (like the one on pages 128–29) and fill it out with these meals. Let the meal plans and recipes in this book inspire you. What did you enjoy during the elimination phase? Did you make up anything new based on new food experiences? Did you have favorite recipes? If you have a go-to list of quick and easy breakfasts, lunches, dinners, and snacks and you always keep the necessary ingredients in your kitchen, then you will never be stuck and faced with a food situation that won't nourish you. These are your fallbacks. Write them down and post them in your kitchen until they become second nature. You'll never say, "I don't know what to eat!" again.

STAY CREATIVE

When you have more time, continue to be creative in your eating. Try making anti-inflammatory versions of your old favorites, remade with better ingredients. When you feel unsure about what to eat, flip through the recipes in chapter 6 for ideas and reminders about what is body-friendly for you. Play with your lists. Be adventurous with vegetables. Expand your culinary horizons.

Some of my patients worry about how to stay firm when they go to restaurants or on vacation or to a party or a friend's house. Nothing has really changed. You are living your life. The only difference is that you now know there are certain foods you are better off not eating. Just let your host or the server know your preferences. Consult your list of foods to avoid. You don't have to make a big deal about it. Bring a dish that you know you can eat to a party. If someone offers you a food you know will cause a problem for you, all you have to do is politely decline.

What really matters, once you are healthy, is that you feed your health most of the time and avoid inflammatory reactors most of the time, whether they are foods or lifestyle habits. Remember that how you live matters, too—how often you move, how much and how well you sleep, how committed you are to connecting to others and having a life purpose. Stay vigilant so you recognize if you begin to slip back into those old inflammatory habits, like sitting too much, staring at screens, withdrawing from social connections, getting caught up in compulsive thoughts or neglecting your passions. Now you know which things are good for *you* and which things aren't. What you pay attention to grows, and what you ignore shrinks, so put your energy into the foods and practices you love—they nurture you, and your health will continue to improve.

STAY THE COURSE

What about "cheating"? My patients ask me about this, too—they worry about being perfect, or what will happen if they have something "forbidden." The concept of cheating, as it relates to food, is antithetical to sustainable wellness. I want you to remember that nothing is forbidden. Everything is a choice. There is a difference between knowing a food is bad for you and choosing not to eat it and forbidding yourself from having a particular food. One is food freedom, and one is food prison. There are no dieting laws here dictating what you can and can't eat. There is no shame here. There is only your health. You want to feel good, so it is logical that you would want to eat what will make you feel good. Eating something that doesn't make you feel good isn't restrictive—it's rational.

But sometimes you will want to do otherwise, and I'll tell you why: temptation, peer pressure, tradition, rituals, old habits, social occasions, family dynamics, and good old-fashioned hedonism. We sometimes consume foods we know we will later regret eating, but the awareness you have gained will make a big difference in how you now perceive those situations. You have knowledge now, so while you still have a choice, now it is an informed and conscious choice, rather than the random eating you used to do before you knew which foods weren't working for your body. You might decide to eat something inflammatory for you, but since you know how you will react, you may decide to have just a little. Or, you may decide that in a given situation, the aftermath will be worth it. *Your decision*, not mine. Not anyone else's.

You may also discover, as your health continues to strengthen, that once in a while, a healthy body may be able to handle a food that isn't good for it. You may discover that a slice of birthday cake or a few potato chips don't throw your health into a tailspin. That's useful knowledge, too. Just beware of dietary drift. Too many compromises in the quality and safety of your food choices can distract you from listening to your body's messages, and that's when your health could start to decline again, as you begin to wander unintentionally away from your own best intentions. If you're not careful, the symptoms can creep back in—and you might not be able to pinpoint which of your foods that cause symptoms is the culprit.

To avoid this, the most important thing you can take from this program is *awareness*. Every time you make a choice about what to eat, every time you don't get enough sleep, every time you get stressed or have a sedentary day or stare at a screen too much or don't reach out to others for connection, notice. Pay close attention to your body's feedback and remind yourself that every bite that goes into your mouth and every action you take for or against your own health is a choice. And of all the choices you make in your day, you probably have the most control over those involving food.

You never, ever have to eat something that will make you feel bad. So what if everyone else is eating it? So what if someone or something—your family, your friends, tradition—dictates that you should eat it? It doesn't have to be a fight. Politely say no and move on to more important things, like conversations, laughter, activities, fun, and living your life.

At first this can feel impossible. Believe me, I know. I remember. You may find yourself thinking things like "But I can't possibly *not* eat cookies at Christmas! I can't possibly avoid pumpkin pie at Thanksgiving! But everyone else wants to order a pizza! It's her birthday/wedding/graduation party, and there's that cake! Halloween candy is practically required, isn't it?"

Remember that these are just echoes of old habits. Of course Halloween candy isn't required, and neither are any of those other things, and you know that. That doesn't mean you *can't* have them, but it also doesn't mean you *have to* have them. You know how your body responds to particular foods, so you can answer these inner questions more rationally, calmly, and with proof to back you up. When you feel tempted to give in, default to that knowledge. If you feel anxious, if you feel deprived, if you feel like you are missing out on something, remind yourself of this truth: Eating food that nourishes your health isn't deprivation. It's one of the most profound of freedoms.

It's the freedom to wake up feeling good every morning—freedom from brain fog, digestive problems, joint and muscle pain, and the life-impeding symptoms of chronic disease. It's the freedom you get in every aspect of your life when your health improves. An inflammation-free life can be yours, and that

> **Eating food that nourishes your health isn't deprivation.**

is much bigger than any fleeting pleasure you might get from eating something inflammatory. But the foods that your body loves, that make you feel great? That's your new jam.

RE-ELIMIN8?

Life happens. Life, as well as bodies and health and biochemistry and bio-individuality, are dynamic, not static. While your intolerances might stay the same, it is always possible that you might develop new ones, and begin to creep back toward the fiery end of the inflammation spectrum. You might not even notice as stress and bad habits sneak back into your life over time. Or, you could develop a health problem despite your best efforts. There are always those factors you can't control that could trigger a health issue. All the more reason to pay attention and make the best possible decisions for your own health—that is how to engineer the best possible outcome for yourself. Most important: Listen to your body.

Paying close attention to the messages from your body will always be the best way to keep track of your current health status, especially as you move through stressful times or experience hormonal transitions such as pregnancy, menopause, or andropause (that's low testosterone, brothers). If you ever find that you have stopped listening for a while—we get busy and overwhelmed and forget to take care of ourselves—bring yourself back to listening to your body's feedback. If you experience any of these life stressors, pay special attention. Has something inflammatory for you crept back in? Bodies change. Time changes us all. Where we are on the inflammation spectrum is always just a snapshot of a moment in time, but over time, that position constantly changes.

If you should ever feel the need, you can always do your elimination program again, to bring down any inflammation that could have crept back in due to whatever may be going on in your life.

Take the quiz in chapter 2 again. You might be having a recurrence in the same category, or you might get completely different results this time. At first maybe your area of dysfunction was digestion or joints and muscles, but now it is your brain or your hormones. If this is the case, do another Core4 or Elimin8 phase of anti-inflammatory living, to help you get back on track.

There are other reasons you may want to do the elimination phase again. Maybe you want to test a new food or try a new dietary strategy, and you want to see if it's right for you. You can always come back as you alter, refine, or perfect your path.

But it's also likely that you may never need the elimination phase again because you now have the tools. You have your foods. You have your lifestyle ideals. And of course, I always encourage you to consult a functional medicine practitioner for an even more personalized program to ferret out any mystery issues you can't solve on your own.

HOW DO YOU FEEL TODAY?

After four or eight weeks of anti-inflammatory living and then a careful reintroduction of selected foods, you should be feeling noticeably better than you did when you started this book. Let's quantify that by reevaluating your health today. Ask yourself:

- How is your energy?

- How is your pain level?

- How are you sleeping?

- How are you concentrating?

- How is your digestion?

- What has changed about your life since you have started this journey?

Now, remember those eight worst symptoms that you originally wrote down on page 54? How does that list look now? Fully resolved? High five! Mostly resolved? Keep exploring, keep testing, keep experimenting, and keep attuned to the messages from your body. It can take a long time for an advanced health imbalance to correct itself, but you are well on your way. When you recognize and name the positive changes in your health, you will have even more motivation for staying true to your newfound knowledge and plan for living.

I also suggest you go back to chapter 2 and take the quizzes again—especially the quizzes where you scored the highest. Now that you have significantly calmed your inflammation and pinpointed your inflammatory foods, your score should be much lower than it was before. Taking the Inflammation Spectrum Quiz again can help you see quantitatively how much you have improved and how much you have moved on the inflammation spectrum toward health and away from chronic disease. That is something to celebrate!

But now that you are headed in the right direction, how do you keep going? Getting inflammatory foods out of your diet has helped clarify your thinking and has worked against any tendency toward food addiction. The inflammatory habits you gave up over the past four or eight weeks have helped calm inflammation by healing your state of mind and your relationship with your body. Targeting your inflammation triggers and getting them out of your diet has helped your body reset, healing your gut and your hormones. You may not feel 100 percent healthy yet, but that's okay, too. In my experience, it can take some people at least six months to completely quell inflammation and heal from its effects, and for many people with health problems it can be up to two years after making significant lifestyle changes that I see meaningful permanent shifts in health status for people experiencing chronic health problems. Wellness is a sacred journey, so be patient and give yourself grace.

Pay attention to your mind, to your feelings about your body and about food. It's all part of the balancing act that is life.

This is the last chapter of this book, but it is the beginning of your next chapter. Your *Inflammation Spectrum* plan has been your springboard for sustainable lifestyle changes based on real information about you. Stay with what your body loves, live your personal life plan, respect what you have learned, steer clear of the things that hurt you, and watch your health continue to improve.

Now that you have a road map for your body, go forward with excitement. What you are doing now is no longer a diet. You know what your body loves and needs to thrive. You have moved from dieter to owner of your own wellness. You know your body better than anyone else ever could—especially now that you have learned how to listen to it.

ACKNOWLEDGMENTS

Amber, Solomon, and Shiloh: My family. I adore you. My heart is walking around outside my body in you three. With every breath, I am yours.

My team: Andrea, Ashley, Yvette, Emily, and Janice. You are part of my family and my closest friends. Thank you for your tireless devotion and passion for the patients we care so much about.

My patients: Thank you for letting me be a part of your sacred journey into wellness. I do not take that responsibility lightly. Serving you is an honor.

Heather, Megan, Marian, Michael, and everyone at Avery and Waterbury: You are the best team I could have dreamed of. Thank you so much for believing in me and for making this book come to fruition.

Eve: This book was our labor of love. Thank you for going on this journey with me.

Jason, Colleen, and my MindBodyGreen family: Thank you for all you have done for me. For giving me a voice and a home over the years. I am eternally grateful.

Elise, Gwyneth, Kiki, and my Goop family: I am immensely grateful for you. Thank you for giving me the chance to share my heart to the world.

Dr. Terry Wahls, Dr. Alejandro Junger, Dr. Josh Axe, and Melissa Hartwig: Thank you for being my heroes, mentors, and friends in this space of wellness and food.

Lee, Jason, Ed, and my Amplify family: Thank you for being my teachers, friends, and core community.

Finally, thank you to everyone in the functional medicine and wellness world: You are world changers.

NOTES

INTRODUCTION

1. Centers for Disease Control and Prevention, "Chronic Diseases in America" infographic, https://www.cdc.gov/chronicdisease/resources/infographic/chronic-diseases.htm.

2. Centers for Disease Control and Prevention, Division for Heart Disease and Stroke Prevention Heart Disease Fact Sheet, https://www.cdc.gov/dhdsp/data_statistics/fact_sheets/fs_heart_disease.htm.

3. World Health Organization Cancer Fact Sheet, http://www.who.int/news-room/fact-sheets/detail/cancer.

4. American Autoimmune Related Diseases Association Autoimmune Disease Statistics, https://www.aarda.org/news-information/statistics/.

5. Andy Menke et al., "Prevalence of and Trends in Diabetes Among Adults in the United States, 1988–2012," *JAMA* 314, no.10 (September 2015): 1021–29. https://jamanetwork.com/journals/jama/fullarticle/2434682.

6. National Institute of Mental Health, Mental Health Information Statistics, https://www.nimh.nih.gov/health/statistics/prevalence/any-mental-illness-ami-among-us-adults.shtml.

7. Centers for Disease Control and Prevention Morbidity and Mortality Weekly Report, https://www.cdc.gov/mmwr/volumes/66/wr/mm6630a6.htm.

8. C. Pritchard, A. Mayers, and D. Baldwin, "Changing Patterns of Neurological Mortality in the 10 Major Developed Countries—1979–2010," *Public Health* 127, no. 4 (April 2013): 357–68; doi: 10.1016/j.puhe.2012.12.018, https://www.ncbi.nlm.nih.gov/pubmed/23601790.

9. Centers for Disease Control and Prevention Autism Spectrum Disorder Data and Statistics, https://www.cdc.gov/ncbddd/autism/data.html.

10. Irene Papanicolas, Liana R. Woskie, and Ashish K. Jha, "Health Care Spending in the United States and Other High-Income Countries." *JAMA* 319, no. 10 (March 13, 2018): 1024–39; https://jamanetwork.com/journals/jama/article-abstract/2674671.

11. Lisa Girion, Scott Glover, and Doug Smith, "Drug Deaths Now Outnumber Traffic Fatalities in U.S., Data Show," *Los Angeles Times*, September 17, 2011; http://articles.latimes.com/2011/sep/17/local/la-me-drugs-epidemic-20110918.

12. Kelly Adams, Martin Kohlmeier, and Steven Zeisel, "Nutrition Education in U.S. Medical Schools: Latest Update of a National Survey," *Academic Medicine* 85, no. 9 (September 2010): 1537–42; https://www.aamc.org/download/451374/data/nutriritoneducationinusmedschools.pdf.

13. Kelly M. Adams, W. Scott Butsch, and Martin Kohlmeier, "The State of Nutrition Education at US Medical Schools," *Journal of Biomedical Education* 2015 (2015), Article ID 357627, 7 pages; http://dx.doi.org/10.1155/2015/357627, https://www.hindawi.com/journals/jbe/2015/357627/.

14. M. Castillo et al., "Basic Nutrition Knowledge of Recent Medical Graduates Entering a Pediatric Residency Program," *International Journal of Adolescent Medicine and Health* 28, no. 4 (November 2016): 357–61; doi: 10.1515/ijamh -2015-0019, https://www.ncbi.nlm.nih.gov/pubmed/26234947.

15. Walter C. Willett et al., "Prevention of Chronic Disease by Means of Diet and Lifestyle Changes," in Dean T. Jamision et al., eds., *Disease Control Priorities in Developing Countries,* 2nd ed. (Washington DC: World Bank Publication, 2006); https://www.ncbi.nlm.nih.gov/books/NBK11795/.

CHAPTER ONE. ANTICIP8

1. L. Cordain et al., "Origins and Evolution of the Western Diet: Health Implications for the 21st Century," *American Journal of Clinical Nutrition* 81, no. 2 (February 2005): 341–54; doi: 10.1093/ajcn.81.2.341, https: www.ncbi.nlm.nih.gov/pubmed/15699220.

2. National Institute of Diabetes and Digestive and Kidney Diseases, Adrenal Insufficiency & Addison's Disease, https://www.niddk.nih.gov /health-information/endocrine-diseases/adrenal-insufficiency-addisons-disease.

3. O. Mocan and D. L. Dumitraşcu, "The Broad Spectrum of Celiac Disease and Gluten Sensitive Enteropathy," *Clujul Medical* 89, no. 3 (2016): 335–42; https://www.ncbi.nlm.nih.gov/pubmed/27547052.

4. E. A. Jeong et al., "Ketogenic Diet-Induced Peroxisome Proliferator-Activated Receptor-Y Activation Decreases Neuroinflammation in the Mouse Hippocampus After Kainic Acid-Induced Seizures," *Experimental Neurology* 232, no. 2 (December 2011): 195–202; https://www.ncbi.nlm.nih.gov/pubmed/21939657.

5. J. Tam et al., "Role of Adiponectin in the Metabolic Effects of Cannabinoid Type 1 Receptor Blockade in Mice with Diet-Induced Obesity," *American Journal of Physiology-Endocrinology and Metabolism* 306, no. 4 (February 15, 2014): E457–68; https://www.ncbi.nlm.nih.gov/pubmed/24381003.

CHAPTER THREE. INCORPOR8

1. Luana Cassandra Breitenbach Barroso Coelho et al. "Lectins, Interconnecting Proteins with Biotechnological/Pharmacological and Therapeutic Applications," *Evidence-Based Complementary and Alternative Medicine* 2017; doi: 10.1155/2017/1594074; https://www.hindawi.com/journals/ecam/2017/1594074/.

2. Lloyd A. Horrocks and Young K. Yeo, "Health Benefits of Docosahexaenoic Acid (DHA)," *Pharmacological Research* 40, no. 3 (September 1999): 211–25; http://www.sciencedirect.com/science/article/pii/S1043661899904954.

3. Kathleen A. Page et al., "Medium-Chain Fatty Acids Improve Cognitive Function in Intensively Treated Type 1 Diabetic Patients and Support in Vitro Synaptic Transmission During Acute Hypoglycemia," *American Diabetes*

Association 58, no. 5 (May 2009): 1237–44; http://diabetes.diabetesjournals.org /content/58/5/1237.short.

4. Puei-Lene Lai et al., "Neurotrophic Properties of the Lion's Mane Medicinal Mushroom, *Hericium erinaceus* (Higher Basidiomycetes) from Malaysia," *International Journal of Medicinal Mushrooms* 15, no. 6 (2013): 539–54; http://www.dl.begellhouse .com/journals/708ae68d64b17c52,034eeb045436a171,750a15ad12ae25e9.html.

5. R. Katzenschlager et al., "*Mucuna pruriens* in Parkinson's Disease: A Double Blind Clinical and Pharmacological Study," *Journal of Neurology, Neurosurgery & Psychiatry* 75, no. 12 (2004): 1672–77; http://jnnp.bmj.com/content/75/12/1672.

6. Ghazala Hussian and Bala V. Manyam, "*Mucuna pruriens* Proves More Effective Than L-DOPA in Parkinson's Disease Animal Model," *Phytotherapy Research* 11, no. 6 (September 1997): 419–23; http://onlinelibrary.wiley.com/doi /10.1002/(SICI)1099-1573(199709)11:6%3C419::AID-PTR120%3E3.0.CO;2-Q/full.

7. Chizuru Konagai et al., "Effects of Krill Oil Containing n-3 Polyunsaturated Fatty Acids in Phospholipid Form on Human Brain Function: A Randomized Controlled Trial in Healthy Elderly Volunteers," *Clinical Interventions in Aging* 8 (September 2013): 1247–57; https://www.ncbi.nlm.nih.gov/pmc/articles /PMC3789637/.

8. Parris Kidd, "Integrated Brain Restoration After Ischemic Stroke—Medical Management, Risk Factors, Nutrients, and Other Interventions for Managing Inflammation and Enhancing Brain Plasticity," *Alternative Medicine Review: A Journal of Clinical Therapeutic* 14, no. 1 (April 2009): 14–35; https://www .researchgate.net/publication/24275478_Integrated_Brain_Restoration_after _Ischemic_Stroke_-_Medical_Management_Risk_Factors_Nutrients_and_other _Interventions_for_Managing_Inflammation_and_Enhancing_Brain_Plasticity.

9. Tracy K. McIntosh et al. "Magnesium Protects Against Neurological Deficit After Brain Injury," *Brain Research* 482, no. 2 (March 1989): 252–60; http://www .sciencedirect.com/science/article/pii/0006899389911888.

10. Inna Slutsky et al., "Enhancement of Learning and Memory by Elevating Brain Magnesium," *Neuron* 65, no. 2 (January 2010): 165–77; http://www .sciencedirect.com/science/article/pii/S0896627309010447.

11. Laura D. Baker et al., "Effects of Aerobic Exercise on Mild Cognitive Impairment: A Controlled Trial," *Archives of Neurology* 67, no. 1 (January 2010): 71–79; https://jamanetwork.com/journals/jamaneurology/fullarticle/799013.

12. Stanley J. Colcombe et al., "Aerobic Exercise Training Increases Brain Volume in Aging Humans," *The Journals of Gerontology: Series A* 61, no. 11 (November 2006): 1166–70; https://academic.oup.com/biomedgerontology/article/61/11 /1166/630432/Aerobic-Exercise-Training-Increases-Brain-Volume.

13. Dietmar Benke et al., "GABA$_A$ Receptors as *in Vivo* Substrate for the Anxiolytic Action of Valerenic Acid, a Major Constituent of Valerian Root Extracts," *Neuropharmacology* 56, no. 1 (January 2009): 174–81; https://www.sciencedirect .com/science/article/pii/S0028390808001950.

14. E. J. Huang and L. F. Reichardt, "Neurotrophins: Roles in Neuronal Development and Function," *Annual Review of Neuroscience* 24 (March 2001): 677–736; https://www.ncbi.nlm.nih.gov/pubmed/11520916.

15. Karl Obrietan, Xiao-Bing Gao, and Anthony N. van den Pol, "Excitatory Actions of GABA Increase BDNF Expression via a MAPK-CREB–Dependent Mechanism—A Positive Feedback Circuit in Developing Neurons," *Journal of Neurophysiology* 88, no. 2 (August 2002): 1005–15; https://www.physiology.org/doi/abs/10.1152/jn.2002.88.2.1005.

16. Pirjo Komulainen et al., "BDNF Is a Novel Marker of Cognitive Function in Ageing Women: The DR's EXTRA Study," *Neurobiology of Learning and Memory* 90, no. 4 (November 2008): 596–603; https://www.sciencedirect.com/science/article/pii/S1074742708001287.

17. S. Parvez et al., "Probiotics and Their Fermented Food Products Are Beneficial for Health," *Journal of Applied Microbiology* 100, no. 6 (June 2006): 1171–85; http://onlinelibrary.wiley.com/doi/10.1111/j.1365-2672.2006.02963.x/full.

18. S. Salminen, E. Isolauri, and E. Salminen, "Clinical Uses of Probiotics for Stabilizing the Gut Mucosal Barrier: Successful Strains and Future Challenges," *Antonie van Leeuwenhoek* 70, no. 2–4 (October 1996): 347–58; https://link.springer.com/article/10.1007%2FBF00395941?LI=true.

19. L. J. Fooks and G. R. Gibson, "Probiotics as Modulators of the Gut Flora," *British Journal of Nutrition* 88, no. S1 (September 2002): s39–s49; https://www.cambridge.org/core/journals/british-journal-of-nutrition/article/probiotics-as-modulators-of-the-gut-flora/0ECB99C9BCC4A6217AA70A51471E3BBA.

20. P. Newsholme, "Why Is L-Glutamine Metabolism Important to Cells of the Immune System in Health, Postinjury, Surgery or Infection?," *The Journal of Nutrition* 131, Supp. 9 (September 2001): 2515S–2522S; https://www.ncbi.nlm.nih.gov/pubmed/11533304.

21. Zhao-Lai Dai et al., "L-Glutamine Regulates Amino Acid Utilization by Intestinal Bacteria," *Amino Acids* 45, no. 3 (September 2013): 501–12; https://link.springer.com/article/10.1007/s00726-012-1264-4.

22. L. Langmead et al., "Antioxidant Effects of Herbal Therapies Used by Patients with Inflammatory Bowel Disease: An *in Vitro* Study," *Alimentary Pharmacology and Therapeutics* 16, no. 2 (February 2002): 197–205; http://onlinelibrary.wiley.com/doi/10.1046/j.1365-2036.2002.01157.x/full.

23. Marta González-Castejón, Francesco Visioli, and Arantxa Rodriguez-Casado, "Diverse Biological Activities of Dandelion," *Nutrition Reviews* 70, no. 9 (September 1, 2012): 534–47; https://academic.oup.com/nutritionreviews/article-abstract/70/9/534/1835513.

24. Marzieh Soheili and Kianoush Khosravi-Darani, "The Potential Health Benefits of Algae and Micro Algae in Medicine: A Review on *Spirulina platensis*," *Current Nutrition and Food Science* 7, no. 4 (November 2011): 279–85; http://www.ingentaconnect.com/contentone/ben/cnf/2011/00000007/00000004/art00007.

25. Ludovico Abenavoli et al., "Milk Thistle in Liver Diseases: Past, Present, Future," *Phytotherapy Research* 24, no. 10 (October 2010): 1423–32; http://onlinelibrary.wiley.com/doi/10.1002/ptr.3207/full.

26. Janice Post-White, Elena J. Ladas, and Kara M. Kelly, "Advances in the Use of Milk Thistle (*Silybum marianum*)," *Integrative Cancer Therapies* 6, no. 2 (June

2007): 104–109; http://journals.sagepub.com/doi/abs/10.1177
/1534735407301632.

27. P. Ranasinghe et al., "Efficacy and Safety of 'True' Cinnamon (*Cinnamomum zeylanicum*) as a Pharmaceutical Agent in Diabetes: A Systematic Review and Meta-analysis," *Diabetic Medicine* 29, no. 12 (December 2012): 1480–92; http://onlinelibrary.wiley.com/doi/10.1111/j.1464-5491.2012.03718.x/full.

28. Haou-Tzong Ma, Jung-Feng Hsieh, and Shui-Tein Chen, "Anti-Diabetic Effects of *Ganoderma lucidum*," *Phytochemistry* 114 (June 2015): 109–13; http://www.sciencedirect.com/science/article/pii/S0031942215000837.

29. L. Liu et al., "Berberine Suppresses Intestinal Disaccharidases with Beneficial Metabolic Effects in Diabetic States, Evidences from in Vivo and in Vitro Study," *Naunyn-Schmiedeberg's Archives of Pharmacology* 381, no. 4 (April 2010): 371–81; https://www.ncbi.nlm.nih.gov/pubmed/20229011.

30. Jun Yin, Huili Xing, and Jianping Ye, "Efficacy of Berberine in Patients with Type 2 Diabetes," *Metabolism* 57, no. 5 (May 2008): 712–17; https://www.ncbi.nlm.nih.gov/pmc/articles/PMC2410097/.

31. Noriko Yamabe et al., "Matcha, a Powdered Green Tea, Ameliorates the Progression of Renal and Hepatic Damage in Type 2 Diabetic OLETF Rats," *Journal of Medicinal Food* 12, no. 4 (September 2009): 714–21; http://online.liebertpub.com/doi/abs/10.1089/jmf.2008.1282.

32. J. Larner, "D-Chiro-Inositol—Its Functional Role in Insulin Action and Its Deficit in Insulin Resistance," *International Journal of Experimental Diabetes Research* 3, no. 1 (2002): 47–60; https://www.ncbi.nlm.nih.gov/pubmed/11900279.

33. F. Brighenti et al., "Effect of Neutralized and Native Vinegar on Blood Glucose and Acetate Responses to a Mixed Meal in Healthy Subjects," *European Journal of Clinical Nutrition* 49, no. 4 (April 1995): 242–47; C. S. Johnston, C. M. Kim, and A. J. Buller, "Vinegar Improves Insulin Sensitivity to a High-Carbohydrate Meal in Subjects with Insulin Resistance or Type 2 Diabetes," *Diabetes Care* 27, no. 1 (January 2004): 281–82; C. S. Johnston et al., "Examination of the Antiglycemic Properties of Vinegar in Healthy Adults," *Annals of Nutrition & Metabolism* 56, no. 1 (2010): 74–79; H. Liljeberg and I. Björck, "Delayed Gastric Emptying Rate May Explain Improved Glycaemia in Healthy Subjects to a Starchy Meal with Added Vinegar," *European Journal of Clinical Nutrition* 52, no. 5 (May 1998): 368–71; M. Leeman, E. Ostman, and I. Björck, "Vinegar Dressing and Cold Storage of Potatoes Lowers Postprandial Glycaemic and Insulinaemic Responses in Healthy Subjects," *European Journal of Clinical Nutrition* 59, no. 11 (November 2005): 1266–71; Nilgün H. Budak et al., "Functional Properties of Vinegar," *Journal of Food Science* 79, no. 5 (May 2014): R757–R764.

34. El Petsiou et al., "Effect and Mechanisms of Action of Vinegar on Glucose Metabolism, Lipid Profile and Body Weight," *Nutrition Reviews* 72, no. 10 (October 2014): 651–61; Brighenti et al., "Effect of Neutralized and Native Vinegar on Blood Glucose and Acetate Responses to a Mixed Meal in Healthy Subjects"; Andrea M. White and Carol S. Johnston, "Vinegar Ingestion at Bedtime Moderates Waking Glucose Concentrations in Adults with Well-Controlled Type 2 Diabetes," *Diabetes Care* 30, no. 11 (November 2007): 2814–15.

35. T. Wolfram and F. Ismail-Beigi, "Efficacy of High-Fiber Diets in the Management of Type 2 Diabetes Mellitus," *Endocrine Practice* 17, no. 1 (January–February 2011): 132–42; https://www.ncbi.nlm.nih.gov/pubmed/20713332.

36. C. L. Broadhurst and P. Domenico, "Clinical Studies on Chromium Picolinate Supplementation in Diabetes Mellitus—A Review," *Diabetes Technology & Therapeutics* 8, no. 6 (December 2006): 677–87; https://www.ncbi.nlm.nih.gov/pubmed/17109600.

37. R. E. Booth, J. P. Johnson, and J. D. Stockand, "Aldosterone," *Advanced Physiological Education* 26, no. 1–4 (December 2002): 8–20; https://www.ncbi.nlm.nih.gov/pubmed/11850323.

38. Z. Lu et al., "An Evaluation of the Vitamin D_3 Content in Fish: Is the Vitamin D Content Adequate to Satisfy the Dietary Requirement for Vitamin D?," *The Journal of Steroid Biochemistry and Molecular Biology* 103, no. 3–5 (March 2007): 642–44; http://www.sciencedirect.com/science/article/pii/S0960076006003955.

39. Joseph L. Mayo, "Black Cohosh and Chasteberry: Herbs Valued by Women for Centuries," *Clinical Nutrition Insights* 6, no. 15 (1998): 1–3; https://pdfs.semanticscholar.org/dcc5/37a8da60cde7b0f5cecb701c2e161b62ac88.pdf.

40. N. Singh et al., "*Withania Somnifera* (Ashwagandha), a Rejuvenating Herbal Drug Which Enhances Survival During Stress (an Adaptogen)," *International Journal of Crude Drug Research* 20, no. 1 (1982): 29–35; http://www.tandfonline.com/doi/abs/10.3109/13880208209083282.

41. Lakshmi-Chandra Mishra, Betsy B. Singh, and Simon Dagenais, "Scientific Basis for the Therapeutic Use of *Withania somnifera* (Ashwagandha): A Review," *Alternative Medicine Review* 5, no. 4 (2000): 334–46; https://kevaind.org/download/Withania%20somnifera%20in%20Thyroid.pdf.

42. L. Schäfer and K. Kragballe, "Supplementation with Evening Primrose Oil in Atopic Dermatitis: Effect on Fatty Acids in Neutrophils and Epidermis," *Lipids* 26, no. 7 (1991): 557–60; https://www.ncbi.nlm.nih.gov/pubmed/1943500.

43. Eric D. Withee et al., "Effects of MSM on Exercise-Induced Muscle and Joint Pain: A Pilot Study," *Journal of the International Society of Sports Nutrition* 12, Supp. 1 (2015): P8, https://www.ncbi.nlm.nih.gov/pmc/articles/PMC4595302/; P. R. Usha and M. U. Naidu, "Randomised, Double-Blind, Parallel, Placebo-Controlled Study of Oral Glucosamine, Methylsulfonylmethane and Their Combination in Osteoarthritis," *Clinical Drug Investigation* 24, no. 6 (2004): 353–63, https://www.ncbi.nlm.nih.gov/pubmed/17516722; Marie van der Merwe and Richard J. Bloomer, "The Influence of Methylsulfonylmethane on Inflammation-Associated Cytokine Release Before and Following Strenuous Exercise," *Journal of Sports Medicine*, https://www.ncbi.nlm.nih.gov/pmc/articles/PMC5097813/.

44. G. S. Kelly, "The Role of Glucosamine Sulfate and Chondroitin Sulfates in the Treatment of Degenerative Joint Disease," *Alternative Medicine Review: A Journal of Clinical Therapeutic* 3, no. 1 (February 1998): 27–39; http://europepmc.org/abstract/med/9600024.

45. Fredrikus G. J. Oosterveld et al., "Infrared Sauna in Patients with Rheumatoid Arthritis and Ankylosing Spondylitis," *Clinical Rheumatology* 28 (January 2009): 29; https://link.springer.com/article/10.1007/s10067-008-0977-y.

46. Kevin P. Speer, Russell F. Warren, and Lois Horowitz, "The Efficacy of Cryotherapy in the Postoperative Shoulder," *Journal of Shoulder and Elbow Surgery* 5, no. 1 (January–February 1996): 62–68; http://www.sciencedirect.com/science/article/pii/S1058274696800322.

47. Barrie R. Cassileth and Andrew J. Vickers, "Massage Therapy for Symptom Control: Outcome Study at a Major Cancer Center," *Journal of Pain and Symptom Management* 28, no. 3 (September 2004): 244–49; http://www.sciencedirect.com/science/article/pii/S0885392404002623.

48. L. Kalichman, "Massage Therapy for Fibromyalgia Symptoms," *Rheumatology International* 30, no. 9 (July 2010): 1151–57; https://www.ncbi.nlm.nih.gov/pubmed/20306046.

49. J. Manzanares, M. D. Julian, and A. Carrascosa, "Role of the Cannabinoid System in Pain Control and Therapeutic Implications for the Management of Acute and Chronic Pain Episodes," *Current Neuropharmacology* 4, no. 3 (July 2006): 239–57, https://www.ncbi.nlm.nih.gov/pmc/articles/PMC2430692/; A. Holdcroft et al., "A Multicenter Dose-Escalation Study of the Analgesic and Adverse Effects of an Oral Cannabis Extract (Cannador) for Postoperative Pain Management," *Anesthesiology* 104, no. 5 (May 2006): 1040–46, https://www.ncbi.nlm.nih.gov/pubmed/16645457.

50. B. Richardson, "DNA Methylation and Autoimmune Disease," *Clinical Immunology* 109, no. 1 (October 2003): 72–79; https://www.ncbi.nlm.nih.gov/pubmed/14585278.

51. Andrzej Sidor and Anna Gramza-Michalowska, "Advanced Research on the Antioxidant and Health Benefit of Elderberry (*Sambucus nigra*) in Food—A Review," *Journal of Functional Foods* 18, Part B (October 2015): 941–58; http://www.sciencedirect.com/science/article/pii/S1756464614002400.

52. Nieken Susanti, "Asthma Clinical Improvement and Reduction in the Number of $CD4^+CD25^+foxp3^+Treg$ and $CD4^+IL-10^+$ Cells After Administration of Immunotherapy *House Dust Mite* and Adjuvant Probiotics and/or *Nigella Sativa* Powder in Mild Asthmatic Children," *IOSR Journal of Dental and Medical Sciences* 7, no. 3 (May–June 2013): 50–59; http://www.iosrjournals.org/iosr-jdms/papers/Vol7-issue3/J0735059.pdf.

53. B. Wang et al., "Neuroprotective Effects of Pterostilbene Against Oxidative Stress Injury: Involvement of Nuclear Factor Erythroid 2-Related Factor 2 Pathway," *Brain Research* 1643 (July 15, 2016): 70–79; https://www.ncbi.nlm.nih.gov/pubmed/27107941.

54. T. Furuno and M. Nakanishi, "Kefiran Suppresses Antigen-Induced Mast Cell Activation," *Biological and Pharmaceutical Bulletin* 35, no. 2 (2012): 178–83; https://www.ncbi.nlm.nih.gov/pubmed/22293347.

55. M. Hatori et al., "Time-Restricted Feeding Without Reducing Caloric Intake Prevents Metabolic Diseases in Mice Fed a High-Fat Diet," *Cell Metabolism* 15, no. 6 (June 6, 2012): 848–60; https://www.ncbi.nlm.nih.gov/pubmed/22608008.

CHAPTER FOUR. INITI8

1. S. Guyenet, "Grains and Human Evolution," *Whole Health Source*, July 10, 2008; http://wholehealthsource.blogspot.com/2008/07/grains-and-human-evolution.html.

2. Oana Mocan and Dan L. Dumitraşcu, "The Broad Spectrum of Celiac Disease and Gluten Sensitive Enteropathy," *Clujul Medical* 89, no. 3 (2016): 335–42; https://www.ncbi.nlm.nih.gov/pmc/articles/PMC4990427/.

3. Jessica R. Biesiekierski and Julie Iven, "Non-Coeliac Gluten Sensitivity: Piecing the Puzzle Together," *United European Gastroenterology Journal* 3, no. 2 (April 2015): 160–65; https://www.ncbi.nlm.nih.gov/pmc/articles/PMC4406911/.

4. Jessica R. Jackson et al., "Neurologic and Psychiatric Manifestations of Celiac Disease and Gluten Sensitivity," *Psychiatric Quarterly* 83, no. 1 (March 2012): 91–102; https://www.ncbi.nlm.nih.gov/pmc/articles/PMC3641836/.

5. S. Lohi et al., "Increasing Prevalence of Coeliac Disease over Time," *Alimentary Pharmacology & Therapeutics* 26, no. 9 (November 1, 2007): 1217–25; https://www.ncbi.nlm.nih.gov/pubmed/17944736.

6. David L. J. Freed, "Do Dietary Lectins Cause Disease?," *BMJ* 318, no. 7190 (April 17, 1999): 1023–24; https://www.ncbi.nlm.nih.gov/pmc/articles/PMC1115436.

7. Pedro Cuatrecasas and Guy P. E. Tell, "Insulin-Like Activity of Concanavalin A and Wheat Germ Agglutinin—Direct Interactions with Insulin Receptors," *Proceedings of the National Academy of Sciences of the USA* 70, no. 2 (February 1973): 485–89; https://www.ncbi.nlm.nih.gov/pmc/articles/PMC433288/.

8. Tommy Jönsson et al., "Agrarian Diet and Diseases of Affluence—Do Evolutionary Novel Dietary Lectins Cause Leptin Resistance?," *BMC Endocrine Disorders* 5 (December 10, 2005): 10; https://bmcendocrdisord.biomedcentral.com/articles/10.1186/1472-6823-5-10.

9. J. L. Greger, "Nondigestible Carbohydrates and Mineral Bioavailability," *The Journal of Nutrition* 129, no. 7 (July 1999): 1434S–1435S; doi: 10.1093/jn/129.7.1434S.

10. I. T. Johnson et al., "Influence of Saponins on Gut Permeability and Active Nutrient Transport in Vitro," *The Journal of Nutrition* 116, no. 11 (November 1986): 2270–77; https://www.ncbi.nlm.nih.gov/pubmed/3794833.

11. Albano Beja-Pereira et al., "Gene-Culture Coevolution Between Cattle Milk Protein Genes and Human Lactase Genes," *Nature Genetics* 35 (November 23, 2003): 311–13; https://www.nature.com/articles/ng1263.

12. S. Pal et al., "Milk Intolerance, Beta-Casein and Lactose," *Nutrients* 7, no. 9 (August 31, 2015): 7285–97; https://www.ncbi.nlm.nih.gov/pubmed/26404362.

13. "New Studies Show Sugar's Impact on the Brain, and the News Is Not Good," *Forbes*, November 8, 2016; https://www.forbes.com/sites/quora/2016/11/08/new-studies-show-sugars-impact-on-the-brain-and-the-news-is-not-good/#337151c1652d.

14. "Latest SugarScience Research," *SugarScience, University of California, San Francisco*; http://sugarscience.ucsf.edu/latest-sugarscience-research.html #.WY4UllGGOkw.

15. Julie Corliss, "Eating Too Much Added Sugar Increases the Risk of Dying with Heart Disease," *Harvard Health Blog*, February 6, 2014; https://www.health.harvard.edu/blog/eating-too-much-added-sugar-increases-the-risk-of-dying-with-heart-disease-201402067021.

16. Kelly McCarthy, "Artificial Sweeteners Linked to Weight Gain over Time, Review of Studies Says," *ABC News*, July 17, 2017; http://abcnews.go.com/Health/artificial-sweeteners-weight-gain-time-review-studies/story?id=48676448.

17. "Dietary Guidelines for Americans Shouldn't Place Limits on Total Fats," *Tufts Now* news release, June 23, 2015; https://now.tufts.edu/news-releases/dietary-guidelines-americans-shouldn-t-place-limits-total-fat.

18. Steven R. Gundry, "Abstract P354: Elevated Adiponectin and Tnf-alpha Levels Are Markers for Gluten and Lectin Sensitivity," *Circulation* 129, Supp. 1 (2018): AP354; http://circ.ahajournals.org/content/129/Suppl_1/AP354.

19. T. Erik Mirkov et al., "Evolutionary Relationships Among Proteins in the Phytohemagglutinin-Arcelin-α-Amylase Inhibitor Family of the Common Bean and Its Relatives," *Plant Molecular Biology* 26, no. 4 (November 1994): 1103–13; https://link.springer.com/article/10.1007/BF00040692#page-1.

20. Richard D. Cummings and Marilynn E. Etzler, "Antibodies and Lectins in Glycan Analysis," in Ajit Varki et al., eds., *Essentials of Glycobiology*, 2nd ed. (Cold Spring Harbor, NY: Cold Spring Harbor Laboratory Press, 2009); https://www.ncbi.nlm.nih.gov/books/NBK1919/.

21. Steven R. Gundry, "Abstract P354: Elevated Adiponectin and Tnf-alpha Levels Are Markers for Gluten and Lectin Sensitivity," *Circulation* 129, Supp. 1 (2018): AP354; http://circ.ahajournals.org/content/129/Suppl_1/AP354.

22. Ibid.

CHAPTER FIVE. ELIMIN8 OR CORE4

1. Environmental Working Group Consumer Guides: www.ewg.org/foodnews/.

2. Keith M. Diaz et al., "Patterns of Sedentary Behavior and Mortality in U.S. Middle-Aged and Older Adults: A National Cohort Study," *Annals of Internal Medicine* 167, no. 7 (October 3, 2017): 465–75; http://annals.org/aim/article-abstract/2653704/patterns-sedentary-behavior-mortality-u-s-middle-aged-older-adults.

3. Christina M. Puchalski, "The Role of Spirituality in Health Care," *Baylor University Medical Center Proceedings* 14, no. 4 (October 2001): 352–57; https://www.ncbi.nlm.nih.gov/pmc/articles/PMC1305900.

4. Ozden Dedeli and Gulten Kaptan, "Spirituality and Religion in Pain and Pain Management," *Health Psychology Research* 1, no. 3 (September 2013): e29.

5. Gaétan Chevalier et al., "Earthing: Health Implications of Reconnecting the Human Body to the Earth's Surface Electrons," *Journal of Environmental and*

Public Health (January 12, 2012): 291541; https://www.ncbi.nlm.nih.gov/pmc /articles/PMC3265077/.

6. "The Health Benefits of Volunteering: A Review of Recent Research," *Corporation for National and Community Service*, 2007; https://www .nationalservice.gov/sites/default/files/documents/07_0506_hbr.pdf.

7. Jacqueline Howard, "Americans Devote More Than 10 Hours a Day to Screen Time, and Growing," CNN, July 29, 2016; https://www.cnn.com/2016/06/30 /health/americans-screen-time-nielsen/index.html.

8. Aviv Malkiel Weinstein, "Computer and Video Game Addiction—A Comparison Between Game Users and Non-Game Users," *The American Journal of Drug and Alcohol Abuse* 36, no. 5 (June 2010): 268–76; http://www.tandfonline .com/doi/abs/10.3109/00952990.2010.491879.

9. Victoria L. Dunckley, "Gray Matters: Too Much Screen Time Damages the Brain," *Psychology Today*, February 27, 2014; https://www.psychologytoday.com /blog/mental-wealth/201402/gray-matters-too-much-screen-time-damages-the -brain.

10. "Prolonged Television Viewing Linked to Increased Health Risks," *Harvard Gazette*, July 6, 2011; http://news.harvard.edu/gazette/story/newsplus /prolonged-television-viewing-linked-to-increased-health-risks/.

11. Julie Taylor, "Are Computer Screens Damaging Your Eyes?," *CNN Health*, November 12, 2013; http://www.cnn.com/2013/11/12/health/upwave -computer-eyes/index.html.

12. Meg Aldrich, "Too Much Screen Time Is Raising Rate of Childhood Myopia," *Keck School of Medicine of USC*, January 22, 2019; http://keck.usc.edu/too-much -screen-time-is-raising-rate-of-childhood-myopia/.

13. Joanne Cavanaugh Simpson, "Digital Disabilities—Text Neck, Cellphone Elbow—Are Painful and Growing," *The Washington Post Health & Science*, June 13, 2016; https://www.washingtonpost.com/national/health-science/digital -disabilities--text-neck-cellphone-elbow--are-painful-and-growing/2016/06 /13/df070c7c-0afd-11e6-a6b6-2e6de3695b0e_story.html?utm_term=.fad03116a6af.

14. Nicholas Carr, *The Shallows: What the Internet Is Doing to Our Brains* (New York: W. W. Norton, 2011).

15. "Body Burden—The Pollution in Newborns: A Benchmark Investigation of Industrial Chemicals, Pollutants, and Pesticides in Human Umbilical Cord Blood," *Environmental Working Group*, July 2005; https://web.archive.org/web /20050716022737/http://www.ewg.org:80/reports/bodyburden2/execsumm.php.

16. James W. Daily, Mini Yang, and Sunmin Park, "Efficacy of Turmeric Extracts and Curcumin for Alleviating the Symptoms of Joint Arthritis: A Systematic Review and Meta-Analysis of Randomized Clinical Trials," *Journal of Medicinal Food* 19, no. 8 (August 2016): 717–29; https://www.ncbi.nlm.nih.gov/pmc /articles/PMC5003001.

17. J. Paul Hamilton et al., "Depressive Rumination, the Default-Mode Network, and the Dark Matter of Clinical Neuroscience," *Biological Psychiatry* 78, no. 4 (August 15, 2015): 224–30; https://www.ncbi.nlm.nih.gov/pmc/articles /PMC4524294/.

18. Shimon Saphire-Berstein et al., "Oxytocin Receptor Gene (*OXTR*) Is Related to Psychological Resources," *Proceedings of the National Academy of Sciences* 108, no. 37 (September 13, 2011): 15118–122; https://www.ncbi.nlm.nih.gov/pm c/articles/PMC3174632/.

19. Lissa Rankin, "Scientific Proof That Negative Beliefs Harm Your Health," *MindBodyGreen*, May 2013; https://www.mindbodygreen.com/0-9690/scientific -proof-that-negative-beliefs-harm-your-health.html.

20. Quora, "This Is What Negativity Does to Your Immune System, and It's Not Pretty," *Forbes*, June 24, 2016; https://www.forbes.com/sites/quora/2016/06 /24/this-is-what-negativity-does-to-your-immune-system-and-its-not-pretty /#421d55e9173b.

21. Lisa R. Yanek et al., "Effect of Positive Well-Being on Incidence of Symptomatic Coronary Artery Disease," *American Journal of Cardiology* 112, no. 8 (October 2013): 1120–25; https://www.ncbi.nlm.nih.gov/pmc/articles/PMC3788860/.

22. Angela K. Troyer, "The Health Benefits of Socializing," *Psychology Today*, June 30, 2016; https://www.psychologytoday.com/blog/living-mild-cognitive -impairment/201606/the-health-benefits-socializing.

23. Eliene Augenbraun, "How Real a Risk Is Social Media Addiction?," *CBS News*, August 22, 2014; https://www.cbsnews.com/news/how-real-a-risk -is-social-media-addiction/.

24. Susan Greenfield, *Mind Change: How Digital Technologies Are Leaving Their Mark on Our Brains* (New York: Random House, 2015).

25. Roxanne Nelson, "Higher Purpose in Life Tied to Better Brain Health," *Reuters*, April 7, 2015; http://www.reuters.com/article/us-stroke-risk-attitude -idUSKBN0MY25Q20150407.

CHAPTER SEVEN. REINTEGR8

1. Isabel J. Skypala et al., "Sensitivity to Food Additives, Vaso-Active Amines and Salicylates: A Review of the Evidence," *Clinical and Translational Allergy* 5 (2015): 34; https://www.ncbi.nlm.nih.gov/pmc/articles/PMC4604636/.

2. Ibid.

3. Jessica R. Biesiekierski et al., "No Effects of Gluten in Patients with Self-Reported Non-Celiac Gluten Sensitivity After Dietary Reduction of Fermentable, Poorly Absorbed, Short-Chain Carbohydrates," *Gastroenterology* 145, no. 2 (August 2013): 320–28.e3; http://www.gastrojournal.org/article/S0016 -5085(13)00702-6/fulltext.

4. M. S. Baggish, E. H. Sze, and R. Johnson, "Urinary Oxalate Excretion and Its Role in Vulvar Pain Syndrome," *American Journal of Obstetrics and Gynecology* 177, no. 3 (September 1997): 507–11; https://www.ncbi.nlm.nih.gov/pubmed /9322615.

INDEX

Page numbers in **bold** indicate charts or tables; those in *italic* indicate figures.

acesulfame K (Sunett, Sweet One), 95
acid reflux, 21, 68, 152, 174, 266
acne, 75, 267
Adaptogenic Adrenal-Balancing
　Smoothie, 249
adaptogens, 248, 251
Addison's disease, 20, 77, 78
adrenal glands, 20, 24, 27, 33, 60, 73, 74,
　75, 77, 78, 126
adzuki, 275
aflatoxin mold, 99
agar, 74
agave nectar/syrup, 58, **84**, 95, 277
age of inflammation, 2–5
albacore tuna, 109
albumin, 60, 64, 102
alcohol, 60–61, 70, 260, 262, 279
aldosterone, 74
alkaloids, 60
allergens/allergies, 246, 260
allspice, 117
almonds, 60, **85**, 101, 262, 274
almond butter, 112, 274
almond milk, 64, 93, 274
alpha-amylase inhibitors, 87
alpha-glucosidase, 72
altar, the benefits of making an, 139
Alzheimer's disease, 3, 67
amaranth, 89, 278
anaphylaxis, 91
anchovies, 109
andropause, 288
animal protein, phasing in, 111
anise, 96
annatto, 117
anthocyanin, 247
antibiotics, 90, 91–92
Anticip8. *See* bio-individuality
anti-inflammatory cookbook,
　192–255, 284
Anti-Inflammatory Turmeric Milk
　(Golden Milk), 251–52

antioxidants, 67, 97, 114, 247, 251, 271
anxiety, 3, 4, 14, 16, 19, 32, 33, 54, 66,
　67, 75, 86, 131, 159, 174, 175, 176,
　177, 268
A1/A2 casein, 92, 269, 276, 277
APOA2/APOE4, 28
apple cider vinegar, 72, 152
applesauce, as egg substitute, 103
apricots, 262
Arctic char, 109
artichokes, 112, 113, 263
artificial sweeteners, 94, 95, 269, 277
arugula, 71, 113
ashwagandha, 75
asparagus, 112, 113, 263
aspartame (Equal, NutraSweet), 95
astaxanthin, 67
asthma, 246
autism spectrum disorders, 3
autoimmune problems, 2, 4, 5, 19, 20,
　24, *25*, 26, 27, 33–34, 66, 68, 75, 77,
　78, 87, 91, 102, 103
autoimmune system (quiz), **47–48**, 49,
　50, 51
Autoimmunity Toolbox, 77–80
autophagy, 81
avocados, 64, 89, 112, 114, 260, 262
avocado oil, 97, 98, 99, 116
Ayurvedic medicine, 66, 75, 254

bacon, 260
baked goods, 88, 89, 102, 278
bananas, 103, 114, 260, 263
banana chips, 102
barley, 57, **84**, 88, 89, 264, 278
barramundi, 109
basil, 117
bass, 109
bay leaf, 117
beans. *See* legumes
Beautifying Blue-Green Mermaid
　Latte, 251

beauty products, natural, 150, 151
beef, 110
beer, 89, 260, 279
beet kvass, 68
beets, 90, 105, 263, 264
beet sugar, 95
behavioral problems, 2, 91
belladonna, 103
berberine, 72
berries, 264
betaine HCL, 69, 111
beverages, 118
BHA and BHT, 97
bike riding, the benefits of, 133
Bio-Individual Inflammation Profile,
    28, 32, 53, 56, 65. *See also*
    Inflammation Spectrum Quiz;
    inflammatory habits; toolboxes
bio-individuality, 1–2, 7, 8, 9, 10–11,
    13–31, 55, 62, 65, 83, 161
bison, 110
bitter greens, 70–71
black beans, 59, **85**, 100, 271, 275
blackberries, 114, 262
black salt, 103
black tea, 262, 276
blenders, high-speed, 246
bloating, 16, 33, 68, 69, 91, 174, 263, 267
blood sugar/insulin system, 24, 25, 32,
    33, 64, 114
blood sugar/insulin system (quiz),
    41–42, 49, *50*, 51
Blood Sugar/Insulin Toolbox, 71–73
blueberries, 102, 114
Blueberry Blast Juice, 247–48
bok choy, 113
bone broth, 118, 260
Bone Broth, Basic, 68, 252–53
bovine growth hormone, 91
brain-adrenal (HPA) axis, 60, 75, 248
brain-derived neurotrophic factor
    (BDNF), 67, 134
brain fog, 16, 32, 66, 67, 106, 268, 287
brain health and fat, 115
brain/nervous system, 23, 32, 34
brain/nervous system (quiz),
    35–36, 49, *50*, 51
Brain/Nervous System Toolbox, 66–67
brain problems, 2, 3, *25*
Brazil nuts, 101
breads, 88, 89
Breakfast-Anytime Nachos, 205–6

Breakfast Steaks with Sweet Potato
    Hash Browns, 219–20
breathing, as substitute for emotional
    eating, 176
brewing your potion, 138
broccoli, 70, 112, 113
broccoli sprouts, 70, 79, 113
bromelain, 246
brown rice syrup, 95
brown sugar, **84**, 94, 95
Brussels sprouts, 70, 103, 112, 113
Brussels Sprouts, Bacon, Apple, and
    Salmon Skillet, 220–21
Buffalo Chicken Dip, 213–14
bulgur wheat, 278
butterfish, 109
butternut squash, 105
butters, **85**, 93, 273, 276
Buttery Garlic-Tarragon Pan-Seared
    Scallops with Shaved Asparagus
    Salad, 232–33
buttery spreads, 98
B vitamins, 70, 79

cabbage, 70, 113, 263
cacao nibs, 97
caffeine, 60–61, 276
calcium, 87
calprotectin, 26
cancers, 2, 5, 131
candy, 95
cane juice, 95
cane juice, evaporated, 95
cane sugar, 58
cannabinoid gene CNR1 rs1049353, 27
cannabis, 76–77
canned food, 260
canola oil, 58, **84**, **85**, 97, 98, 270, 278
cantaloupe, 114
caraway, 117
carbonated water, 118
cardamom, 117
carob/carob powder, 97, 263
carrots, 90, 105
casein, 57, 90, 91, 92–93, 269, 276, 277
cashews, 60, 101, 260, 263, 274
cashew butter, 274
cashew milk, 93
cassava, 90, 102, 103
catfish, 109
cauliflower, 70, 113, 263
Cauliflower-Broccoli Tabbouleh, 226

Cauliflower-Nut Flatbreads, 214
Cauliflower-Walnut Tacos, 206–7
cayenne pepper, 104, 275
CBD oil, 76–77
celery, 113, 177
celery seed, 117
celiac disease (CD), 20, 34, 77, 78, 85
cellphone elbow, 141
cereals, 88, 96
chard, 70, 113
chasteberry, 74
cheese, 57, **84**, 91, 92–93, 93–94, 260, 277
chemical air fresheners, 150, 151
cherries, 102, 262
chestnuts, 101
chia seeds, **85**, 101, 273
chicken, 110
Chicken and Vegetable Lo Mein,
    233–34
chicken sausage, 103
Chicken Zoodle Soup, 227
chickpeas, **85**, 112, 260
chili peppers, 275
chili powder, 104
Chili-Spiced Nuts and Cranberries, 215
chives, 113
chlorella, 112
chocolate, 260
Chocolate, Coconut, and Hemp
    Energy Balls, 215–16
cholesterol, 32, 73, 115–16
chondroitin sulfate, 76
Chopped Kale Salad with Thai
    Peanut Dressing, 199–200
chromium, 73
chronic diseases, 2
chronic inflammation, 23
cilantro, 70, 117
cinnamon, 72, 96, 117, 246–47
citrus fruits, 260
clam, 109
Clean Fifteen, 113
cleaning your home, the benefits
    of, 149, 151
clean protein, 108–11
clementines, 114
clove, 117
cocoa, 264
coconuts, 64, 96, 97
Coconut–Butternut Squash
    Porridge, 193
coconut cream, 194, 211, 213

coconut flakes or shreds, 102
coconut kefir, 68, 80
coconut milk, 64, 93, 94, 101, 241
coconut oil, 66, 97, 98, 99, 116, 150–51, 262
coconut sugar, 58, **84**, 95, 269, 277
coconut water, 118, 263
cod, 109
coffee, 276
coffee creamer, 57
cognitive function. *See* brain/nervous
    system
Cole, Will, 1–11
    drwillcole.com, 265
    Ketotarian, 9, 10, 61, 81, 115
    See also Inflammation Spectrum
collagen powder, 76
collard greens, 71, 89, 113
"compliant" ingredients, 192
computer vision syndrome, 141
concentration problems, 32, 66, 268
congestion, 259, 267
constipation, 33, 54, 68, 252, 263, 267
cooking, oils and fats for, 99, 116
cooling inflammation and healing,
    106–91
Core4
    overview of, 56–58, 60, 63, 64, 83, **84**,
        119–20, 156, 258
    reintegrating foods, 269–70, 273
    repeating, 288–89
    See also elimination diet;
        Inflammation Spectrum Quiz
Core4 and Elimin8 (Elimination
    Phase), 29, 83
    Day 1: grains, 85–90
    Day 2: dairy products, 90–94, 101
    Day 3: added sweeteners, 94–97
    Day 4: inflammatory oils, 97–99
    See also Elimin8 (Elimination Phase)
Core4 and Elimin8 (healing)
    food lists (what to eat), 106,
        108–19, 283
    pre-week prep steps, 107, 121, 126
    sample meal plans, 107, 121–26, **122–25**
    schedule
        Week 1:, 127–33, **128–29**
        Week 2: 134–43, **136–37**
        Week 3: 144–52, **146–47**
        Week 4: 153–61, **154–55**
    See also Elimin8 (healing)
Core4 (recipes), 121, 192, 193–218.
    See also elixirs and broths

coriander, 117
corn, 57, **84**, 88, 89, 269, 278
corn oil, 58, **84**, **85**, 97, 98, 270, 278
corn sugar/syrup, 9, 58, **84**, 94, 95, 269, 277, 279
cortisol, 75, 159
cottonseed oil, 98
crab, 109
cravings, 32, 95, 96, 135, 257–58
crawfish/cray fish, 109
Cre8. *See* designing your new, personalized food and life plan
C-reactive protein, 26
cream, **84**, 91, 93, 276, 277
Creamy Coconut-Ginger Squash Soup, 235
creativity in eating, 284–85
croaker (fish), 109
cross-reactivity labs, 27
Crunchy Roasted Chickpeas, 216–17
Crunchy Veggie Rolls with Homemade Ranch Dressing, 240–41
cryotherapy, 76
cucumbers, 113
cumin, 117
curcumin, 76, 246
currants, 102
curry powder, 104

dairy products, 57, 59, 62, 64, **84**, 90–94, 263, 269, 276
dandelion tea, 70
dates, 262
date sugar/syrup, 58, 95, 269, 277
D-chiro-inositol, 72
decorating with natural materials, the benefits of, 151
Dedic8. *See* anti-inflammatory cookbook
default meals, 284
deglycyrrhizinated licorice, 69
deli salads, 96
dementia, 26, 66
depression, 2–3, 4, 16, 19, 32, 66, 67, 85, 175, 268
designing your new, personalized food and life plan, 282–91
desserts, 95–96
detoxification system, 24, 25, 33
detoxification system (quiz), 39–40, 49, 50, 51
Detoxification Toolbox, 69–71

diabetes, 2, 5, 19, 20, 33, 71, 72, 78, 88, 94, 141
diamine oxidase (DAO) enzyme blockers, 261–62
diarrhea, 33, 68, 91, 252, 263, 267
diets, 14–15, 30
diet sodas, 95
digestion system (quiz), **37–38**, 49, *50*, 51
digestion problems, 4, 19, 23, 25, 32, 33, 34, 103, 106, 114, 259, 260, 262, 263, 267, 271, 287
Digestion Toolbox, 68–69
digestive enzymes, 69, 111
dill, 117
Dilled Smoked Salmon–Cucumber Bites, 241–42
Dirty Dozen, 113
disease management, 3–4, 6, 18–19, 20
docosahexaenoic acid (DHA), 66
dopamine, 66
Dr. Will Cole's Gut-Healing Smoothie, 249
Dressing, Thai Peanut, 199–200
dried fruits, 96, 262
drug use, 70
drwillcole.com, 265
dry brushing, 71
dry skin, 33, 267
duck, 110
dulse, 74, 113

earthing, the benefits of walking barefoot in sand, grass, or dirt, 139
eating disorders, 30
eating out, 173–74, 284
eating without viewing a screen, 143
edamame, 64, 100, 271, 276
eggs, 60, 62, 63, 64, **85**, 89, 102–3, 270, 274
egg substitutes, 103
egg-free breakfasts, 102, **124**
Egg-Free Mayonnaise, 230
eggplant, 60, **85**, 87, 104, 260, 262, 275
einkorn, 89
elderberry, 79
Elimin8
    overview of, 56, 58–60, 63, 83, 84, **84–85**, 119, 156, 258
    reintegrating foods, 270–71, 273
    repeating, 288–89
    See also elimination diet; Inflammation Spectrum Quiz

Elimin8 (Elimination Phase)
  Day 5: legumes, 99–100
  Day 6: nuts and seeds, 100–102
  Day 7: eggs, 102–3
  Day 8: nightshades, 103–5
  See also Core4 and Elimin8
    (Elimination Phase)
Elimin8 (healing)
  Mid-Elimin8 Track Checkpoint, 157,
    161–62
  schedule
    Week 5: 162–69, **164–65**
    Week 6: 169–77, **170–71**
    Week 7: **180–81**, 178–84
    Week 8: 185–91, **186–87**
  See also Core4 and Elimin8 (healing)
Elimin8 (recipes), 121, 192, 219–45.
    See also elixirs and broths
elimination diet, 7–11, 23–25, 28, 29, 30,
    34, 53, 119, 130. *See also* Core4;
    Elimin8
Elimination Phase, 83–105, 256,
    258, 259
elixirs and broths, **122**, **124**, 126, 138,
    246–55
elk, 110
emotional disorders, 2
emotional eating, stress eating,
    as inflammatory habit, 121,
    174–77
emu oil, 79
endive, 113, 262
endocannabinoid system, 27
endocrine system. *See* hormonal
    system
energy drinks, 95, 262
Environmental Working Group, 113
environment tolerance and
    bio-individuality, 17
enzyme inhibitors, 87, 88
epigallocatechin-3-gallate
    (EGCG), 72
epigenetics, 13
erectile dysfunction, 116
esophageal damage, 68
estrogen, 74
evening primrose oil, 75
exercise, 17, 67, 127, 134, 144, 153, 163,
    172, 178–79, 185
extra-virgin oils, 98, 116
extra-virgin cod-liver oil, 79
eye irritation, 267

fatigue, 4, 16, 19, 21, 91, 106, 268
fats, 64, 88, 94, 110, 115–16. *See also*
    inflammatory oils
fatty liver disease, 70
fava beans, 100
fear of missing out (FOMO), 182, 183
feeling, reevaluating, 289–91
fennel, 117
fenugreek, 117
fermented foods, 68, 80, 260, 276, 278
ferritin, 26
fever, 268
fiber, 73, 88, 271
fibromyalgia, 33, 75
Fig and Olive Tapenade, 242–43
flaxseeds, 101, 273
flounder, 109
flours, grain-free, 90, 103
Fluffy Grain-Free Pancakes, 193–94
flu-like symptoms, 16
focus problems, 66, 268
FODMAPs, 259, 260, 263–64,
    280, 283
folate, 70, 247
food allergies, intolerances,
    sensitivities, 7, 8, 15–16, 145, 288
food as medicine, 5, 6–7, 15, 21, 65
food confusion to food freedom, 10.
    See also Inflammation Spectrum
food pyramid, 85
forest bathing (*shinrin-yoku*), 131–32
free-writing, the benefits of, 177
friend time, the benefits of, 167
fruit, 64, 88, 96, 114–15, 263, 264
fruit drinks, bottled, 95
fruit juice, 95, 264
fruit juice, concentrated, 95
functional medicine, 4–7, 10, 14, 18–19,
    20–21; 26, 32, 78, 259, 265, 289

GABA, 67
Galangal Broth, 69, 253–55
gallbladder, 33, 69, 70, 115
garbanzo beans, 100
garlic, 70, 117, 264
Garlicky Butternut Squash Noodles
    with Kielbasa, 199
gas, 69, 91
genetics, 1, 9, 13, 14, 15, 19, 21, 22, 23, 27,
    28, 66, 99
ghee, 93, 97, 99, 116
gherkins, 262

ginger, 113, 117, 247, 251–52, 254
Ginger-Garlic Shrimp and Cabbage,
    207–8
giving yourself a gift, the benefits
    of, 189
glucosamine sulfate, 76
gluten, 87, 88, 264, 278
gluten sensitivity, 27, 85
gluten-free grains, 269, 278
goji berries, 60, 104, 114
Goldilocks principle, 23
gonadal axis, 73
Good Health score, 52, 52
goose, 110
grains, 57, 59, 62, 64, **84**, 85–90,
    263, 269, 278
granola bars, 96
grapefruit, 114, 260
grapes, 262
grapeseed oil, 58, **84**, **85**, 98
gratitude, the benefits of expressing,
    185, 188
Graves' disease, 78
green beans, 100, 264
green juices, 118
green olives, 262
Green Queen Juice, 247
Greens and Herbs, Lemony Fish Soup
    with, 227–28
Greens and Hummus Breakfast Bowl,
    194–95
green smoothies, 89
green tea, 60–61, 262, 276
Guacamole-Stuffed Baby Bells, 217
guavas, 262
gut autoimmunity, 77
"gut feeling," 69
Gut-Soothing Ginger and Slippery
    Elm Tea, 248–49

habits. *See* inflammatory habits;
    specific habits
ham, 260
hash, breakfast, 103
Hashimoto's thyroiditis, 34, 78
hazelnuts, 60, 101, 274
hazelnut milk, 93, 274
HCL, 248
healing and inflammation, 22–23
healing and cooling inflammation,
    106–91
health care system, 3–4, 6, 18–19, 20

Health Problems score, 52, 52
heartburn, 33, 54, 152, 267
heart problems, 2, 5, 16, 19, 20, 26, 94,
    115, 141, 267
heavy metals, 70
hemp, 76–77
hemp milk, 273
hemp seeds, 101
hempeh, 111
hempfu, 64
HEPA filters, 151
herbs, 96, 97, 116–17
herbal teas, 96, 97, 276
Herb-Crusted Cauliflower Steaks with
    Mushroom-Onion Scramble, 221–22
herring, 109
hickory nuts, 101
hidradenitis suppurativa, 78
high blood pressure, 32
high-fructose fruit, 263, 264
high-fructose corn syrup, 9, **84**, 94, 95,
    269, 277, 279
histamines, 252, 259, 260–61, 280, 283
hives, 91, 267
holy basil (tulsi), 158
Homemade Ranch Dressing, 241
homestretch, 156–57
homocysteine, 26
honey, 58, **84**, 95, 262, 264, 269, 277
honeydew melon, 114
hormonal problems, 4, 19, 24, 33, 87, 116
hormonal system (quiz), 43–44, 49, 50, 51
Hormone (Endocrine System) Toolbox,
    73–75, 249
horseradish, 117
houseplants, the benefits of, 151
hsCRP (high-sensitivity C-reactive
    protein), 26
Hummus and Greens Breakfast Bowl,
    194–95
hypothalamic-pituitary-adrenal (HPA)
    axis, 60, 73, 75, 248

ice cream, 57, 91, 92–93, 93
IL-6 (interleukin 6), 26, 135
immune system. *See* autoimmune
    system
immunity and bio-individuality, 17
Incorpor8. *See* Core4; Elimin8;
    toolboxes
inducible nitric oxide synthases
    (iNOS), 79

indulgences, 106, 131–32, 139–40,
148–49, 157–58, 167, 173–74, 182,
189, 284
industrial farming, 85
Inflammation profile. *See* Bio-
Individual Inflammation Profile
Inflammation Spectrum, 1–11, 19–30
anti-inflammatory cookbook,
192–255, 284
bio-individuality, 1–2, 7, 8, 9,
10–11, 13–31, 32, 55, 56, 62, 65,
83, 161
cooling inflammation and healing,
106–91
designing your new, personalized
food and life plan, 282–91
elimination diet, 7–11, 23–25, 28, 29,
30, 34, 53, 119, 130
elimination phase, 83–105, 256,
258, 259
lab tests for, 25–28
stepping down process, 29, 56, 57, 58,
84–85, 84–105
testing your old favorites, 29–30, 60,
88, 108, 179, 191, 256–81
See also Cole, Will; Inflammation
Spectrum Quiz; inflammatory
habits
Inflammation Spectrum Quiz, 24, 28,
34–53, 65, 289, 290. *See also*
Bio-Individual Inflammation
Profile; Core4; Elimin8;
Inflammation Spectrum
inflammatory habits, 2, 7, 8, 10, 29, 31,
57, 59, 106, 107, 119–21, 127, 134, 144,
156, 163, 172, 179, 185, 285, 290. *See
also* Bio-Individual Inflammation
Profile; Inflammation Spectrum;
lifestyle; *specific habits*
inflammatory oils, 58, 59, **84**, **85**, 97–99,
269–70, 277–78, 279. *See also* fats;
oils (healthy)
infrared sauna, 76
Initi8. *See* Elimination Phase
insulin. *See* blood sugar/insulin
system
insulin resistance, 71, 72, 88, 131
interacting with people, the benefits of,
142–43
interleukin 6 (IL-6), 26, 135
intermittent fasting (IF), the benefits
of, 81

*International Journal of Adolescent
Medicine and Health,* 5
intestinal permeability, 26
intestinal ulcers, 68
inulin (sugar alcohol), 264
Investig8. *See* Bio-Individual
Inflammation Profile
iron, 26, 79, 87, 247, 264
irritable bowel syndrome (IBS), 16, 34,
68, 69, 78, 263
isomalt (sugar alcohol), 264
itching, rashes, 16, 33, 267

jicama, 113
Jicama Fish Tacos, 236–37
joint pain, 16, 25, 32, 33, 34, 54, 75, 76,
91, 103, 246, 260, 268, 271, 287
joy of missing out (JOMO), 183
juicers, 246
juniper/juniper berry, 117
junk foods, 9

kale, 70, 90, 102, 113, 247, 264
Kamut, 89
kefir, 68, 80, 260, 276, 277
kefiran, 80
kelp, 74, 113
Ketotarian (Cole and Will), 9, 10,
61, 81, 115
kidney beans, 100
kidneys, 24, 33, 69, 264
kimchi, 68, 260
kiwifruit, 114
kohlrabi, 113
kola nuts, 101
kombu, 74, 113
kombucha, 68, 118, 260
krill oil, 67

labels, the importance of reading, 92,
95, 96, 98, 103, 110, 192
lab tests, 25–28
lack of higher purpose, as
inflammatory habit, 121, 189–91
lactoferrin, 26
lactose, 57, 90, 91, 92–93
lamb, 110
Latte, Beautifying Blue-Green
Mermaid, 251
laughing more, the benefits
of, 160
lavender, 117

L-dopa, 66
leafy greens, 70–71
leaky blood-brain barrier, 26, 32, 66
leaky gut syndrome, 32, 33, 66,
    68, 87, 252
learning something new,
    the benefits of, 190
lectins, 59–60, 62, 63, 64, 87, 88, 99,
    100, 275
leeks, 113
Legs-up-the-Wall Pose (yoga), 148–49
legumes, 59–60, 62, 63–64, 65, **85**, 87,
    99–100, 260, 263, 264, 271, 275
lemons, 114, 247, 260, 264
lemon balm, 117
Lemon-Thyme Parsnip Fries, 243
Lemony Fish Soup with Herbs and
    Greens, 227–28
lentils, 59, 65, **85**, 100, 111, 271, 275
letter writing and mailing, the benefits
    of, 184
lettuce, 113
lettuce wraps, 89
L-glutamine, 69
licorice root, 69
lifestyle, 5, 6, 10, 11, 13, 21–25, 29, 57, 59,
    61, 179, 282, 289, 290, 291. *See also*
    inflammatory habits
lima beans, **85**, 100
limes, 114, 260, 264
lion's mane mushroom, 66
lipopolysaccharides (LPS), 26, 66, 87
liqueur, 279
listening to music, the benefits of, 157,
    176, 182
listening to your body, 130, 157, 172,
    179, 185, 188, 267, 269, 286, 288, 291
live events, the benefits of
    attending, 143
liver, 24, 33, 60, 69, 70–71, 71–72, 94, 114,
    115, 152, 277
lobster, 109
lupus, 34, 75, 78, 103
Lyme disease, 70
lymphatic system, 24, 33, 69, 70, 71, 139

macadamia nuts, 101, 274
maca powder, 112
mace, 117
mackerel, 74, 109
magnesium, 247
magnesium glycinate, 67, 158

mahimahi, 109
maltitol (sugar alocol), 264
Mango Tuna Salad–Stuffed
    Popovers, 201
mannitol (sugar alcohol), 264
mantras, 67, 69, 71, 73–75, 75–77,
    80, 81, 127, 134, 135, 144–45, 153,
    156, 163, 185
maple sugar/syrup, 58, **84**, 95, 269, 277
margarines, 98
massage, the benefits of, 76, 139–40, 182
mastitis, 91, 92
matcha (green tea), 72
mayonnaise, 102–3, 202, 230
Mayonnaise, Basic Homemade, 202
MCT oil, 66
meal plans, forms, **128–29**, **136–37**,
    146–47, **154–55**, **164–65**, **170–71**,
    180–81, **186–87**, 284
meal plans, sample, 107, 121–26,
    122–25
meditation, 67, 77, 127, 131, 134, 135, 138,
    144–45, 153, 156, 157, 158, 162, 163,
    169, 172, 178, 185
melons, 264
memory problems, 32, 66, 67, 116, 268
menopause, 73, 75, 288
menstruation problems, 33
mercury in fish, 108, 110
meringue, 102
metabolic syndrome, 33, 71, 88
metformin, 72
methylation, 27, 70, 79
methylsulfonylmethane (MSM), 76
Mexican Avocado Baked Eggs, 195–96
microbiome, 14, 26, 248
Mid-Elimin8 Track Checkpoint, 157,
    161–62
migraines, 10, 13, 16, 67, 267
milk, 57, **84**, 90, 91, 92–93, 93, 101, 277
milk thistle, 70
millet, 89, 278
mindful awareness, 159, 160, 167,
    168, 286
minerals, 79
mint, 117
miso, 100, 276
mold, exposure to, 70
monkey mind (racing thoughts), 121,
    167–68, 175
monk fruit, 58, **84**, 95, 277
mood changes, 32, 33, 66, 73, 259, 268

morning glories, 103
MTHFR (methylation-gene
    mutation), 27
mucuna pruiens (kapikacchu), 66
multiple autoimmune-reactivity labs,
    26–27
multiple sclerosis (MS), 20, 77, 78
multitasking, 132
mung beans, 65, 100, 111, 271, 275
muscle pain, 16, 32, 268, 287
musculoskeletal system, 24, 25, 33
musculoskeletal system (quiz), **45–46**,
    49, *50*, 51
Musculoskeletal Toolbox, 75–77
mushrooms, 100, 114, 260, 264
mushroom caps, 89
muskmelon, 114
mussels, 109
mustard, 117
mustard greens, 71
My Eight Worst Symptoms Right Now,
    54, 161, 259, 290

napping, the benefits of, 157, 177
natto (fermented soy), 63, 64, 111, 276
natural sweeteners, 94, 95, 269, 277
naturally sweetened foods, 96–97
nature, the benefits of spending time
    in, 131–32, 142, 143
nausea, 267
navy beans, 100
negativity, as inflammatory habit, 121,
    158–60
neoroplasticity, 67
nerve growth factors (NGFs), 66
neurological autoimmunity, 77
neurological problems, 20, 91, 259,
    260, 262
neurotransmitters, 66, 67, 260
neutral food, the idea that no
    foods are, 6
NF-kB proteins, 79
nightshade vegetables, 60, **85**, 87, 103–5,
    114, 262, 271, 275
nondairy yogurt, cheese, ice cream, 93
nori, 74, 114
Nrf2 pathway, 79
nutmeg, 117
nutritional yeast, 102, 103, 112
nutrition education, 5
nuts and seeds, 60, 62, 63–64, 65, **85**, 87,
    93, 100–102, 260, 270, 273

nut butters, 274
Nuts, Seeds, and Coconut Granola, 196

oats, 57, 88, 89, 278
obesity, 3, 71
occludin (gut-lining protein), 26
oils (healthy), 115–16. *See also*
    inflammatory oils
oils, cold-pressed, 97, 98, 116
oil diffuser, essential, 138
okra, 114
olives, 64, 114
olive oils, 64, 97, 98, 99, 116, 262
omega-3 fatty acids, 66, 88
omega-6 fatty acids, 75, 88
"one thing that finally helped," the
    fallacy of believing in, 14–15
onions, 70, 264
"optimism gene," 158
oranges, 114, 260, 262
oregano, 117
organic meat/poultry, 110
organics, prioritizing, 112–13
organ meats, 79
orthorexia, 30
osteoarthritis, 75
osteoporosis, 87
ostrich, 110
outside, using natural products, 151
oxalates, 259, 264–65, 280, 283
oysters, 109

palm oil, 66
palm shortening, 99, 116
pancreas, 24, 33, 115
Pan-Seared Flounder with Kohlrabi,
    Carrot, and Apple Slaw, 237–38
Pan-Seared Salmon on Bitter Greens
    with Sweet Cherries, 208–9
papayas, 114
paprika, 104, 275
Parkinson's disease, 66
parsley, 70, 117
passion fruit, 114
pasta, 88, 89
PCOS (polycystic ovary syndrome), 75
peanuts and peanut products, 59, **85**,
    99, 100, 260, 264, 275
peanut butter, **85**, 275
Peanut Thai Dressing, 199–200
peas, 100, 112, 264
pecans, **85**, 101, 274

peppercorn, 117
peppers, 60, **85**, 87, 104, 262, 275
"perfect diet," the fallacy of believing in the, 9
perimenopause, 73–74
pernicious anemia, 78
personality and bio-individuality, 17
personal life plan, 282–84
Pesto-Stuffed Chicken Breasts with Chunky Tomato Sauce, 209–10
pets and walking, the benefits of, 133
pharmaceutical drugs, side effects of, 4, 18
phosphatidylcholine, 67
phosphatidylserine, 67
phosphorus, 247
phytic acid/phytates, 60, 62, 63, 64, 87, 88, 99
pico de gallo, 105
pili nuts, 101, 112
pimientos, 104
pineapple, 114, 246, 262
pine nuts, 101
pinto beans, 59, 65, **85**, 100, 271, 275
pistachios, 101, 274
plantains, 90, 102
plant-based cheese, milk, 93–94
plant-based protein, 111–12
plant-centric diet, adapting to a, 61, 62, 63
plant fats, 64
playing active game with kids, 133
plums/prunes, 262
PMS, 73, 75
polenta, 278
pollock, 109
pollutants, exposure to, 21
polyinflammation, 24, 25, 34
polyinflammation assessment (quiz), 49, 50, 51, 53
Polyinflammation Toolbox, 80–81
polyunsaturated fatty acids, 97
Poor Health score, 52, 52
poppy seeds, 101
pork, 110
positivity, the benefits of, 158, 159, 160
potatoes, 60, **85**, 87, 103–4, 262, 275
Power Greens Smoothie, 222
prediabetes, 2, 33, 71, 88
pregnancy, 288
premature death, 131, 141
prescription drugs, 3–4, 6, 18–19, 20, 70

pressure cookers, the benefits of cooking with, 63–64, 65, 68, 275
proanthocyanidins, 72
probiotics, 69
processed foods, 95, 98, 100, 192, 260, 271
produce, 112–15
progesterone, 74
prolonged sitting, as inflammatory habit, 120, 131–33
Prosciutto Chips, Three Ways, 244
protease inhibitors, 87
protein, 108–11, 247, 271
protein powders, 100
psoriasis, 78
pterostilbene, 79
Pumper-Upper Treg Smoothie, 250
pumpkin, 103, 105
pumpkin seeds, 60, **85**, 101

quail, 110
Quick Dal with Cauliflower Rice, 202
Quick Veggie Pickles, 244–45
quinoa, 57, **84**, 87, 88, 89, 269, 278

rabbit, 110
radishes, 114
rainbow trout, 109
raspberries, 115
reactions to food or influences, measuring, 267–79, 272–73, **280**
rebooting your body, 130
recipes, 192–255, 284
red beans, 100
red clover blossom, 70
red pepper flakes, 104
refined sugars, 94
Refreshing Adrenal-Balancing Iced Tea, 248–49
refried beans, 100
Reintegr8. *See* testing your old favorites
reintegration plan, 265–66, 273–79
Reintegration Test Worksheet, 272, **280**, 280–81, 283
reishi mushrooms, 72
Rejuvenating Celery Juice, 248
repetitive thoughts, Stanford University study on, 158
resveratrol, 79
rheumatoid arthritis, 34, 75, 78, 103
rhubarb, 114, 115
riboflavin, 247
rice, 88, 89, 269, 278

rice bran oil, 98
Roasted Pork Chops with Olives and Grapes, 238–39
roasting, industrial seed oils, 100–101
rooibos tea, 75
root vegetables, 96, 102, 105
Root Vegetable Curry, 211
rosemary, 117
runny nose, 16
rutabaga, 100, 114
rye, 57, **84**, 87, 88, 89, 264, 278

saccharin (Sweet'N Low), 95
sacha inchi, 101, 111
safflower oil, 98
safflower seeds, 101
sage, 117
salami, 260
salicylates, 259, 262, 280, 283
salmon, 74, 109, 260
Salmon, Beet, and Shaved Fennel Salad, 228–29
salsa, 105
sandwiches, 85, 89, 103, 203
saponins, 87
sardines, 74, 109
saturated fats, 28
sauerkraut, 68, 260, 264
Sausage-Stuffed Apples, 222–23
scallions, 114, 264
scallops, 109
schisandra powder, 75
scleroderma, 78
screen staring, as inflammatory habit, 120, 140–43
seafood, 108–9
sea salt, 117
sea vegetables, 74
seaweed, 114
sesame seeds, 60, **85**, 101
sex drive (low), 33, 73, 116
Sex-Hormone Boosting Elixir, 250
shellfish, 260
showering, the benefits of vigorous scrubbing and using moisturizer, 176
shrimp, 109
Shrimp, Bacon, and Okra with Garlicky Cauliflower Grits, 224–25
Shrimp Cakes with Creamy Dilled Slaw, 229–30
silent autoimmunity, 78

"sitting is the new smoking," 131
Sjögren's syndrome, 75, 78
Skin-Brightening Lavender Tonic, 251
skin problems, 16, 32, 33, 34, 75, 85, 91, 103, 259, 260, 262, 267, 271
skipjack tuna, 109
sleeping more, the benefits of, 157–58
sleep problems, 268
slippery elm powder, 69
slip-ups, cheating on your dietary plan, 107–8, 161–62, 285–88
small intestinal bacterial overgrowth (SIBO), 68, 260
smoked meat products, 260
Smoked Salmon Salad, 203
snacks, 101, 113, 115, 121, **123**, **125**, 175, 213–18, 240–45, 270, 278–79, 284
Snack-Size Italian Meatballs, 245
snow peas, 100
soaking legumes, nuts and seeds, 63, 76, 118–19, 273, 274, 275
social isolation and/or social media addiction, as inflammatory habit, 121, 182–84
socializing and bio-individuality, 17
social life, the benefits of having a, 166
sodas, 95
sole, 109
Sole Water, 74
sorbitol (sugar alcohol), 264
South American–style "nachos," 90
soy, 58, 59, 63, 64, 100, 264, 271, 275, 276
soybeans, **85**, 99, 260
soybean oil, **84**, **85**, 98, 270
sparkling water, 97
spay day, 182
spelt, 57, 87, 88, 89, 264, 278
spices, 97, 117, 273, 275
Spiced Beef Burgers with Sweet-and-Sour Red Cabbage, 239–40
Spiced Mushroom and Veggie Hash with Sunshine Eggs, 197
spinach, 70, 112, 114, 260, 265
spinach pesto, 209
spirits (vodka, rum, whiskey, tequila), 279
spiritual practice, the benefits of, 135, 138–39, 190
spirulina, 70, 112, 251
sports, the benefits of joining in, 133, 163
sprouts (alfalfa, bean, broccoli, etc.), 114

squash, 87, 102, 114
squid (calamari), 109
standing desks, the benefits of, 132
star anise, 117
starchy vegetables, 100
starting doing something you used to
    love but stopped doing, the
    benefits of, 190
staying the course, 26, 107–8, 135, 153,
    161–62, 169, 172–73, 179, 188, 285–88
Steak and Carrot Noodle Bowl with
    Chimichurri Sauce, 230–31
stepping down process, 29, 56, 57, 58,
    84–85, 84–105
stevia, 58, **84**, 95, 277
stomach pain, 16, 33, 69, 91, 263
stomach ulcers, 68
strawberries, 115, 260
stress, 21, 73, 75, 120, 159, 288
stress eating, 121, 174–77
stress tolerance and bio-
    individuality, 17
sucralose (Splenda), 95
sugar, 88, 277
sugar alcohols, 58, **84**, 95, 264, 277
suicide, 2–3
sulforaphane, 70, 79
sulfur-containing vegetables, 70
sumac, 117
sunflower oil, 58, **84**, **85**, 98
sunflower seeds, 60, **85**, 101
supplements, 65
sweeteners, added, the problem
    with, 58, 59, **84**, 92, 94–97, 263,
    269, 277, 279
sweeteners, hidden, 96
sweet potatoes, 90, 96, 100, 103, 104,
    105, 265
Sweet Potato BLTs, 203–4
Sweet Potato Breakfast Skillet, 198
Sweet Potato–Date Smoothie, 225
Swiss chard, 114, 265
symptoms, after elimination phase,
    259–65
symptoms, inflammation upstream
    from, 22
systemic lupus erythematosus, 78
systems medicine. *See* functional
    medicine

tamari, 276
tangelos, 115, 262

tangerines, 262
T-cell function, 79
teas, 60–61, 70, 75, 96, 97, 118, 262, 276
tempeh, 63, 64, 100, 111, 276
testing your old favorite foods and
    habits, 29–30, 60, 88, 108, 179, 191,
    256–81
testosterone issues, 73
text neck, 141
Thai ginger, 254
Thai Peanut Dressing, 199–200
THC, 77
theater, the benefits of attending
    live, 143
thiamine, 247
thinking about the future, 179
thinning hair, 33
thyroid problems, 34, 73, 74
Thyroid-Boosting Smoothie, 249–50
tigernuts, 102
tilapia, 109
time-restricted feeding (TRF), 81
toast with avocado slices, 103
tobacco, 104
tofu, 64, **85**, 100, 271, 276
tomatillos, 60, 104
tomatoes, 60, **85**, 87, 103–4, 260, 262, 275
tomato sauce, 275
toolboxes, 8, 28, 29, 31, 51, 55, 56, 65–82,
    83, 126, 127, 134, 144, 153, 162, 172,
    178, 185, 246. *See also* Bio-
    Individual Inflammation Profile
"toxic" feeling, 70
toxin exposure, as inflammatory habit,
    120, 149–52
tracks, 56–65. *See also* Core4; Elimin8
trans fats, 58
travel breaks, the benefits of taking, 132
Treg Pumper-Upper Smoothie, 250
triggers, inflammation downstream
    from, 22, 290
triggers for negativity, 160
triglycerides, 72, 73
Tropical Spice Juice, 246–47
tuna, 109
turkey, 110
turmeric, 76, 117, 152, 246
turnips, 100, 114
type 1 diabetes, 78
type 2 diabetes, 33, 71, 72, 88

USDA MyPlate, 85

valerian root, 67
vanilla bean, 117
vegetables
    cooked vs. raw, 68
    fermented, 68
    FODMAPs and, 263
    grains vs., 88
    high-fiber, 73
    nightshade, 60, **85**, 87, 103–5, 114,
        262, 271, 275
    root, 96, 102, 105
    sea, 74
    starchy, 100
    sulfur-containing, 70
vegetable chips, 90
vegetables chips, roasted, 102
vegetable oils, 58, **84**, **85**, 97, 98, 270
vegetable soup, 103
vegetarians and vegans, 61–65, 99, 111
Veggie-Avocado Mash Coconut
    Wraps, 232
venison, 110
vinegar, 260
vitamins, 79, 247
vitamin D, 74
vitamin K$_2$, 79, 80
vitiligo, 78
volunteering, the benefits of, 139, 191

wakame, 74
Waldorf Salad Wrap, 204–5
walking, the benefits of, 127, 132–33,
    143, 176
walnuts, 60, **85**, 101, 260, 274
walnut butter, 274
watching a funny show,
    the benefits of, 177

water, 118, 177
water, retaining, 268
water chestnuts, 114, 262
water kefir, 68, 80
weak nails, 33
week-by-week walk-through, 107,
    127–91
Weeknight Beef Pho, 212
weight problems, 4, 21, 32, 33, 54, 106,
    130, 268
weight training, 134, 163
weighing yourself, the benefits of
    stopping, 145, 172, 188
wheat, 57, **84**, 87, 88–89, 263, 264
whey, 91
white beans, 59, **85**, 100, 271, 275
whitefish, 109
white sugar, **84**, 94, 95
white tea, 60–61, 276
"wild-caught" fish, 66, 74, 99, 110
windows, opening, the benefits
    of, 151
wine, 260, 279

xenobiotics, 91
xylitol (sugar alcohol), 58, 95, 264, 277

yams, 96
yellowfin tuna, 109
yerba maté, 262
yogurt, 57, 64, **84**, 91, 92–93, 93, 96, 260,
    276, 277

Zone of False Wellness, 52, 52
zonulin (gut-lining protein), 26
Zucchini Hummus Cucumber Sushi
    Rolls, 218

Also by DR. WILL COLE

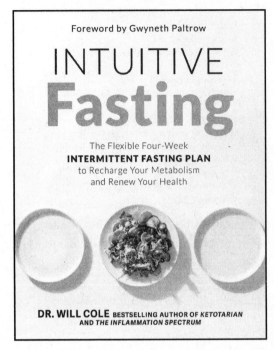

Get in touch with your instinctive eating patterns to reset your body, recharge your metabolism, renew your cells, and rebalance your hormones.

🌱
RODALE

A new twist on keto: the fat-burning power of ketogenic eating meets the clean green benefits of a plant-centric plate.

AVERY

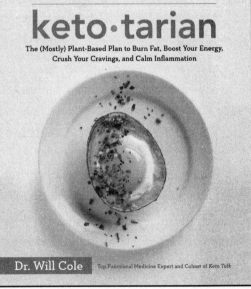

ABOUT DR. WILL COLE

Dr. Will Cole, DC, IFMCP, a leading functional medicine expert, graduated from Southern California University of Health Sciences. His extensive postdoctoral education and training is in functional medicine and clinical nutrition. Dr. Cole consults with people around the world via webcam at www.drwillcole.com and locally in Pittsburgh, Pennsylvania. He specializes in clinically investigating underlying factors of chronic disease and customizing health programs for thyroid issues, autoimmune conditions, hormonal dysfunctions, digestive disorders, and brain problems.

Dr. Cole was named one of the top fifty functional medicine and integrative doctors in the nation. A charismatic and popular TV guest, frequently called upon to offer advice on health issues, Dr. Cole is a national speaker on functional medicine topics and is a health expert and course instructor for MindBodyGreen and Goop, two of the largest wellness websites in the world, for which he has written hundreds of articles and led popular video classes. Dr. Cole has also written and been featured in popular articles for *Vogue*, *Bustle*, and *Reader's Digest*.

Dr. Cole has also received extensive training in the biological sciences—anatomy, physiology, pathophysiology, epidemiology, histology, blood chemistry, neurology, and pharmacology—as well as conventional medical diagnosis, clinical nutrition, botanical medicine, and lifestyle counseling. He is committed to finding root causes rather than treating symptoms with drugs. His focus is to promote health and optimal function through natural, noninvasive methods such as nutritional therapy, herbs, supplements, stress management techniques, and lifestyle changes.